M000281850

Dr. Ian Smith's
Guide to Medical Websites

IAN K. SMITH, M.D.

DR. IAN SMITH'S GUIDE TO MEDICAL WEBSITES

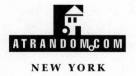

NEW YORK

Library of Congress Cataloging-in-Publication Data
Smith, Ian K. (Ian Kenneth).
Dr. Ian Smith's guide to medical websites.
p.   cm.
ISBN 0-8129-9181-8 (pbk. : alk. paper)
1. Medicine—Computer network resources. 2. Medical care—Computer
network resources. 3. Communication in medicine. 4. Internet. I. Title:
Doctor Ian Smith's guide to medical websites. II. Title: Guide to
medical websites. III. Title.
R859.7.E43 S64   2001   025.06′61—dc21   2001046000

Website address: www.atrandom.com
Printed in the United States of America on acid-free paper
2   4   6   8   9   7   5   3

First Edition

Contents

How to Use This Guide

Every week my e-mail box is full of thousands of requests for medical information from readers of my columns in *Time* magazine and the New York *Daily News,* and from viewers of my reports on NBC's *Today* show and WNBC-TV in New York City. Most of their questions concern where on the Internet they can find websites that will provide them with accurate and current information about a specific medical condition.

I have often wished in the past that I had a reference to recommend, but there really isn't any convenient book that rates the thousands of sites I have encountered that offer medical information. Since I spend so much of my time on the Internet using websites to research diseases, it simply made sense to me that I could use my vast experience and write the book myself.

There are thousands of medical websites on the Internet that offer everything from specific advice to research findings, but there is no real classification system that tells consumers the reliability of the information or the credentials of the sources providing the information. The website listings in this book represent what in my judgment are the best health websites on the Internet. With a few exceptions, I have excluded retail sites or sites that are sponsored by private companies, in an attempt to collect sources providing the most impartial information available.

This book is organized alphabetically by various areas of medical specialty. You can also refer to the Index at the back of the book to find sites pertaining to your medical concern. To further help you navigate these sites, I've provided a paragraph about each site and ranked them on a scale of one to three (three represents the highest rating) according to the following criteria:

- **Source.** This rating represents my assessment of the expertise of the source of information and also reflects the frequency of updates to the information.
- **Navigation.** This rating reflects my judgment of the ease with which information can be found on the site and the efficiency of the search function of the site.
- **Interactivity.** This rating is based on my analysis of the extent to which a visitor can obtain personal answers to questions, use tables and calculators to get specific information, and the quality and number of links within the text to other relevant articles or websites.
- **Overall.** The overall rating is based on the cumulative ratings in the three categories above and represents my overall assessment of the total look and feel of the site.

It is my hope that this book provides you with the knowledge and informed medical information you need to participate with your physician in caring for your health and the health of those you love. The Internet is a powerful tool that can be extremely helpful in understanding medical information. Use it wisely and judiciously and you will reap the potential benefits.

Dr. Ian Smith's
Guide to Medical Websites

The Top Ten
General Medical Websites

About.com
www.about.com

One of the greatest collections of information on diseases and conditions on the Net. It spans the globe and provides interactive chats and forums for experts and patients to come together. This site not only directs you to outside sources, but also takes each topic and gives you the rundown from top to bottom.

Best Doctors
www.bestdoctors.com

The idea behind this site is simple: find the best doctors and provide the best content on a site that others can access free of charge. Founded by a man who was diagnosed with an inoperable tumor and wanted the best doctors to treat him, he set out to empower other patients through information.

HealthAtoZ.com
www.healthatoz.com

This is the kind of site that contains so much information that there's little chance you won't find what you're looking for. Not only are the diseases covered extensively, but the interactive tools make your search for information much more enjoyable. Come here to learn, then take advantage of links to other sources to intensify your search for information.

Healthcommunities.com
www.healthcommunities.com

This site is specifically designed to give you disease-related information through what it calls channels. It's one of the most interactive medical portals on the Net, offering chats, discussion forums, and clinical trials. This site enables you to access the world of medicine in seconds.

healthfinder
www.healthfinder.gov

This government portal opens the world of Internet medicine. Whether it's through tools such as libraries, online journals, or medical dictionaries or hot topics that might interest you, this site delivers quickly and with reliability. A big bonus of the site is that it also provides content in Spanish.

InteliHealth
www.intelihealth.com

It's important for a portal to "have it all." This one is a good example. Whether it's drug information, a medical dictionary, or a rundown on a long list of diseases and conditions, Intelihealth is your gateway to top-notch information. It doesn't hurt to have Harvard Medical School's consumer health information tied to the site.

MedicineNet.com
www.medicinenet.com

You don't have to be a member to access this deep site of medical information. Other than listing every disease known to man, this site offers a built-in medical dictionary that will help you distinguish between tendons and ligaments and allow you to follow more closely those phrases thrown about on NBC television's hit, *ER*.

National Institutes of Health
www.nih.gov

This is arguably the leading collection of health research institutes in the world. Whether the topic is allergy and infectious disease or cancer, this is your gateway to health information. You'll find the latest in research and well-written fact sheets and brochures that reach out to inform us all.

National Library of Medicine
www.nlm.nih.gov

This is the best electronic medical library in the world. It gives you access to the most important research and links to thousands of sites, sending you around the globe for the best information in a matter of seconds. Physical medical libraries, beware—this site could one day put you out of business!

WebMD
www.webmd.com

One of the most heavily marketed portals on the Net, this site stands up to most of the hype. It's nicely divided for different audiences, ranging from patients and doctors to physician assistants to health teachers. It has a robust television service that allows you to watch broadcasts on different health topics.

Acne

Absolute Acne Info
www.absoluteacneinfo.com

Source: 1
Navigation: 2
Interactivity: 1
Overall: 1

Because of the blinking ad that greets you immediately, you might think this site lags when it comes to content. Not so. You have to do a bit of searching, but eventually you will find informed and useful answers to questions regarding acne. There aren't many places where you'll read about acne psychology. You will also read about some of the natural treatments that some patients have tried and hear from practitioners in the skin community center. You'll find out about treatments and facts that will explode many of those acne myths.

Acne Canada
www.acnecanada.com

Source: 3
Navigation: 3
Interactivity: 1
Overall: 2

Here's a great site about acne from north of the border. Although you might have to click more than you'd like to get to the information you want, it's worth it. The definitions and descriptions are concise. And it's easy to follow along with the content. Its credentials are impeccable, as health care providers assist in its operation.

Acne-Care.com
www.acne-care.com

Source: 1
Navigation: 3
Interactivity: 1
Overall: 1

Here you'll find general definitions of acne and how to go about treating it. The site also deals with many of the myths surrounding acne. There's nothing outstanding about this site, but it's easy enough to navigate and deals satisfactorily with the topic.

Acne.net
www.acne.net

Source: 3
Navigation: 1
Interactivity: 1
Overall: 1

This is a useful site with regard to acne. It's a very basic yet functional website. There's nothing fancy, but it's effective. You do have to scroll down to the FAQs section to really get to the meat of the information, such as treatment and myths.

Acne-Site
www.acne-site.com

Source: 1
Navigation: 3

Interactivity: 1
Overall: 1

This is a good eclectically sourced site. It's as though some of the best information from other sites has been cut and pasted here saving time. The site's fairly easy to navigate and has interesting information on prescription drugs used to fight acne. It's not too detailed, but there is enough information to satisfy basic queries.

American Academy of Dermatology
www.aad.org/pamphlets/acnepamp.html

Source: 3
Navigation: 3
Interactivity: 1
Overall: 3

This is an online pamphlet by the AAD. The information is general and basic yet thorough. There's really nothing to click on, as you just scroll down from one topic to another. Explanations are concise and to the point. You won't be overwhelmed with clinical terminology.

AcneNet
www.skincarephysicians.com/acnenet

Source: 3
Navigation: 3
Interactivity: 1
Overall: 2

Right on the first page you'll find a link to the most common and basic questions regarding acne. Myths are cleared up here, and real treatments are prescribed. Simple to navigate, the site also has enough content to satisfy. The focus is on teen acne, but adult acne sufferers will also find helpful information.

Dermatology Channel
www.dermatologychannel.net/follicle/acne

Source: 3
Navigation: 3
Interactivity: 3
Overall: 3

Could a site be easier to use while providing such good content? Everything you need to know about acne and how to treat it is here. From traditional treatments to alternative ones, it's all considered. It's sophisticated enough for adults, yet simple enough for teenagers.

MEDLINEplus on Acne
www.nlm.nih.gov/medlineplus/acne.html

Source: 3
Navigation: 3
Interactivity: 1
Overall: 3

This website includes information from other sources. As with other MEDLINEplus subject headings, all of it is useful. This page is dedicated solely to acne, and its strength lies in the store of information gathered from elsewhere and placed under one umbrella. In essence, it's a search engine of sorts. Here you can also find some resources for Spanish speakers.

National Institute of Arthritis and Musculoskeletal
   and Skin Diseases
www.nih.gov/niams/healthinfo/acne/acne.htm

Source: 3
Navigation: 3
Interactivity: 1
Overall: 2

This site is essentially a fact sheet and a great quick reference: simple, straightforward, and effective. It's a one-stop shop for information on acne. Just point and click to have your general questions on acne answered. It couldn't be any easier to navigate.

Adolescent Health
See **Teen Health, General.**

AIDS
See **HIV/AIDS.**

Allergies

Allergy Society of South Africa
www.allergysa.org/allsa.htm

Source: 2
Navigation: 3
Interactivity: 1
Overall: 2

This site of the Allergy Society of South Africa is one of the best organized and most informative on the Internet. Its home page is colorful, easy to navigate, and full of internal and external links that will make your search for information very smooth. There's a kid's corner that will tell you about the disease in children, as well as a link to diagnostic tests. While the society doesn't vouch for the tests, many are commonly used and quite helpful. You can keep track of your allergies online and turn the information in to your physician on the next visit.

American Academy of Allergy, Asthma and Immunology
www.aaaai.org

Source: 3
Navigation: 2
Interactivity: 1
Overall: 2

This site could provide all you need to know about allergies. It has the best science and research behind it, something that is evident in its thorough fact sheets and excellent links. The site contains a huge amount of information, but you can get whatever you want quickly. Check out the Allergy Report while you're there. The tips section, also offered in Spanish, can help you keep your nose dry and your airways open. If you need to consult an allergist, the physician referral service might be helpful.

American College of Allergy, Asthma & Immunology
    Online
www.allergy.mcg.edu

Source: 3
Navigation: 3

Interactivity: 3
Overall: 3

If you want reliable, easy-to-access information on allergies, this is your site. You will be treated to excellent information on the basics as well as what's in store from the research labs. The interactivity of this site is amazing. You can take an allergy quiz or locate an allergist near you, and kids can take asthma tests. The site has something for everyone whether you are a consumer, a journalist, or a doctor. In spite of an unfortunate link to a pharmaceutical company on the home page, this is a superb site. Be sure to visit this site and visit it often.

Asthma and Allergy Foundation of America
www.aafa.org

Source: 3
Navigation: 3
Interactivity: 2
Overall: 3

This is one of my favorite allergy sites for consumers and professionals. The information is plentiful, and the site is organized in a way that invites you to search for more. There are extensive links to other websites and Net resources. You can also ask an allergist a question and read other questions and answers that have been posted. This site will not leave you wanting more.

Food Allergy and Anaphylaxis Network
www.foodallergy.org

Source: 3
Navigation: 3
Interactivity: 1
Overall: 2

If you suffer from food allergies or just want to learn more about them, surf no more. This site is put together by the American Academy of Allergy, Asthma and Immunology, the National Association of Nurses, and the American Dietetic Association. The information is extremely reliable, comprehensive, and easy to understand. A great feature is a link to the Kids and Teen food allergy sites. They are equally informative and tremendously helpful.

HealthAtoZ.com on Allergies
www.healthatoz.com/atoz/allergies/allergyindex.html

Source: 2
Navigation: 3
Interactivity: 2
Overall: 2

This is one of the most complete and credible allergy websites you'll find. It has an enormous amount of information, and if you have a fancy for alternative medicine, it's here for the taking. There are several interesting interactivity features, including checking the pollen count and finding your nearest allergist. With just a few clicks, you'll discover how to fight allergies naturally or which are the sneeziest U.S. cities. You can't go wrong by visiting this site.

Joint Council of Allergy, Asthma, and Immunology
www.jcaai.org

Source: 3
Navigation: 3
Interactivity: 1
Overall: 2

This is not for the beginner looking for allergy information. There is excellent information on a wide range of allergy-related issues, but if you don't know the basics, it might not be helpful. The newsletter and the practice guidelines are wonderful sources of information, but what you take away from them will depend on your level of understanding of allergies and the immune system. Give it a try—at the very worst, you can click on to the links it lists.

MayoClinic.com Allergy & Asthma Center
www.mayoclinic.com/home?id=3.1.1

Source: 3
Navigation: 2
Interactivity: 2
Overall: 2

This site is where to go for no-frills, tell-it-as-it-is information on allergies. The renowned Mayo Clinic is one of the most trusted and respected authorities in the world, and this website reflects its high standing in the medical community. The information center addresses all of the major issues involving allergies. Once you're done reading that, go to the interactive section and try the personal health scorecard.

National Institute of Allergy and Infectious Diseases
www.niaid.nih.gov

Source: 3
Navigation: 1
Interactivity: 1
Overall: 2

This is the home of the U.S. government's service on allergy and infectious diseases. The information, as you would expect, is current, thorough, and well written. Allergy fact sheets and graphics make learning the information quite easy. There's a section of news releases that highlight the latest research. While the site offers few links, the ones it does are exceptional, so trying them could complete your circle of knowledge.

> World Allergy Organization—IAACI
> www.worldallergy.org
>
> *Source: 3*
> *Navigation: 3*
> *Interactivity: 1*
> *Overall: 2*

This site belongs to an international allergy organization that provides important and credible information to health care professionals as well as patients. Get an allergy update or use some of the great resources to find information on other sites. You can sign up to receive the e-letter on allergy news or find out which organizations might help you obtain more allergy information. Come here to get connected elsewhere.

Alternative Medicine
See site list in Web Resources Directory, p. 239.

Alzheimer's Disease

> Ageless Design
> www.agelessdesign.com/alz.htm
>
> *Source: 1*
> *Navigation: 2*
> *Interactivity: 3*
> *Overall: 1*

Information on age-related conditions such as Alzheimer's and Parkinson's diseases. There are a free newsletter, news services, and an "ask the expert" option (though the credentials of the experts are not provided). It seems very useful and has a somewhat more homemade feel than more typical medical websites—but the credibility and foundation of the content are not readily apparent.

The Alzheimer Page
www.biostat.wustl.edu/alzheimer

Source: 1
Navigation: 3
Interactivity: 1
Overall: 1

This site belongs to Washington University, St. Louis, one of the leading medical and research institutions in the world. It has loads of information from Alzheimer's basics to family support. You can read questions others have asked about caring for Alzheimer's patients; though the answers aren't from medical experts, they come from many who have had long experience. This is a site that might best serve you by allowing you to read about the experiences of others and accessing the links to other sites that discuss the illness.

Alzheimer Research Forum
www.alzforum.org

Source: 3
Navigation: 3
Interactivity: 1
Overall: 2

A site with easy-to-read and -understand information about Alzheimer's disease, as well as a substantial number of outside

resources and references listed. A Scientific Advisory Board
corroborates the information, and the site is certainly easy to
navigate. The "Ethical Issues" section is uncommonly interesting. The best place to visit on this site is the "General Information" section: www.alzforum.org/public/layperson_sites.html

Alzheimer's Association
www.alz.org

Source: 3
Navigation: 3
Interactivity: 2
Overall: 3

This is a great place to increase your understanding about
Alzheimer's disease, learn about recent advances in science
and public policy, and locate the Alzheimer's Association chapter nearest you. Highly credible, easy to navigate, and overall
an impressive site for an association—very informative and
user-friendly, not just self-promoting or soliciting members. A
good place to browse.

Alzheimer's Disease Education and Referral (ADEAR)
    Center
www.alzheimers.org

Source: 3
Navigation: 3
Interactivity: 3
Overall: 3

A highly credible service provided by the National Institute on
Aging (NIA) that provides information about Alzheimer's disease and information on other resources. The name of the center and its site couldn't be more perfect—it's a top-notch

education and referral resource for those seeking information on Alzheimer's. A toll-free number is listed for visitors who want to speak with an "information specialist" to answer any questions. A multimedia section provides educational audio and video segments. It's not a pretty site—but it is pretty useful.

Alzheimer's Disease International
www.alz.co.uk

Source: 3
Navigation: 3
Interactivity: 1
Overall: 3

Alzheimer's Disease International (ADI) is an umbrella organization of Alzheimer's associations around the world that offer support and information to people with dementia and their caregivers. The section "Help for Caregivers" (www.alz.co.uk/caregivers) is where all information for patients and caregivers can be found—it's not the best name for the section—and really is the bulk of the site.

AlzheimerSupport.com
www.alzheimersupport.com

Source: 1
Navigation: 2
Interactivity: 3
Overall: 1

This is a less sophisticated website in its tone and appearance. The overwhelming e-commerce orientation detracts from the health educational feel of the site; however, many visitors may be interested in the products as well as the information. It does provide several community features for patients and caregivers, such as message boards, chat rooms, doctor referral suggestions, and support group listings by geographic area that will be e-mailed to you on request. It's a good place to stop for information and products, but don't make it your only stop in the road to information on or support for people dealing with Alzheimer's disease.

American Health Assistance Foundation
www.ahaf.org/alzdis/about/adabout.htm

Source: 3
Navigation: 3
Interactivity: 2
Overall: 2

The American Health Assistance Foundation (AHAF) is a nonprofit charitable organization with more than twenty-five years dedicated to funding research and educating the public on Alzheimer's disease, glaucoma, macular degeneration, heart disease, and stroke. The AHAF also provides emergency financial assistance to Alzheimer's disease patients and their caregivers. It is an excellent resource for patients and caregivers, and, although the site solicits funds, its primary focus is clearly providing education, resources, and services for its visitors.

CBS HealthWatch on Alzheimer's Disease
www.cbshealthwatch.medscape.com/alzheimerscenter

Source: 3
Navigation: 3

Interactivity: 2
Overall: 2

A top-notch consumer health site that covers every major health condition. In spite of the commercial look of the site due to heavy advertising, you'll find excellent background information about Alzheimer's disease, feature articles for the newly diagnosed as well as more knowledgeable patients and caregivers, current news, FAQs, an "ask the expert" option, community features, a wealth of resources and searches through the library, related links, and much more. This is an excellent site for many conditions and can be a great starting point to learn more about Alzheimer's and where to go for more detailed information.

Center for Mental Health Services
www.mentalhealth.org/search/DoSearch.asp; search for
   "Alzheimer's"

Source: 3
Navigation: 2
Interactivity: 1
Overall: 2

This website, a service of the U.S. Department of Health and Human Services, is organized by disease areas. This is obviously not a complete website for Alzheimer's disease, but it is an important site for the more knowledgeable patient or caregiver to check out. The DHHS has compiled a short but informative list of news and articles on the condition, with sources including the National Institute of Mental Health, the Agency for Health Care Policy and Research (AHCPR), the National Institutes of Health, and the Administration on Aging, to name a few. You won't find customized tools or resources or a place to ask questions, but you'll get the current Alzheimer's facts from leading medical institutions.

> National Institute of Neurological Disorders and
>   Stroke/Alzheimer's Disease Information Page
> www.ninds.nih.gov/health_and_medical/disorders/
>   alzheimersdisease_doc.htm
>
> *Source: 3*
> *Navigation: 3*
> *Interactivity: 2*
> *Overall: 2*

This is really an Alzheimer's fact sheet rather than an entire website by the NINDS of the NIH; however it is worthy of inclusion in our list as it is highly credible, is very easy to read, and provides other valuable resources. The NIH is always a good resource for health topics, and therefore this page is included in our list. A quick reference for other resources.

Arthritis

> American College of Rheumatology
> www.rheumatology.org
>
> *Source: 3*
> *Navigation: 3*
> *Interactivity: 1*
> *Overall: 3*

It's not surprising that the country's foremost rheumatology organization has produced one of the Internet's best rheumatology websites. The information on these pages is credible, abundant, and written for all to understand. You will learn more than you ever expected about arthritis and its related diseases. Also, the site links you to other Internet resources—not that you'll really need them after devouring this site's information!

Arthritis Canada
www.arthritis.ca

Source: 2
Navigation: 3
Interactivity: 1
Overall: 2

This is one of Canada's best web offerings on arthritis. No, the home page is not in French, but if that's what you prefer, the information is offered in that language also. The site provides information for everyone, whether you're a patient or an orthopedic surgeon. Just click on the "Patients" link, and you'll find more information than you probably anticipated. On the home page there's also a list of other arthritis websites that you can access with a simple click. This is a must stop on your quest for arthritis info.

Arthritis Foundation
www.arthritis.org

Source: 3
Navigation: 3
Interactivity: 2
Overall: 3

When I'm searching for information on arthritis, this is usually where I begin. The site is well organized, and it doesn't take too many clicks to find exactly what you want. Click on "Disease Center," and a long list of the different types of arthritis pops up on-screen. Then take your choice. I've never been let down by this site. The information is accurate and easy to read. Whether you're a patient looking for treatment information or a doctor looking for the latest research, this is the place to go. You can also look at the message boards and read the experiences of other patients and physicians.

Arthritis News on the Net
www.cancernews.com/arthritis

Source: N/A
Navigation: N/A
Interactivity: N/A
Overall: 1

This is not your site if you want to access arthritis information with just one click. Instead, it is a site full of links to other arthritis resources from books, magazine articles, and the latest headlines. When you've exhausted other resources and want a quick method of finding more Internet information, this is where you want to go.

Arthritis Research Campaign
www.arc.org.uk

Source: 2
Navigation: 3
Interactivity: 1
Overall: 2

This British site tackles arthritis efficiently and thoroughly. It's neatly organized into sections, including "about arthritis" and "news and views." These are the two places where you'll want to stop and absorb all of the well-written information about the different types of arthritis. I hadn't discovered this site until I was writing this guide, but you better believe that now it's been added to my list of favorites.

Focus on Arthritis
www.focusonarthritis.com

Source: 2
Navigation: 3
Interactivity: 2
Overall: 2

This is a busier site, but the information is easily found on the home page or is just two clicks away. Physicians contribute a lot of this information, so its credibility level is high. You can get the latest headlines here, as well as the ABCs on the arthritic conditions. Because there's so much here, you might not need to visit many other sites. There's an entire "Community" section that includes support groups and message boards—something here for everyone.

Hospital for Special Surgery Rheumatology Division
www.rheumatologyhss.org

Source: 3
Navigation: 2
Interactivity: 1
Overall: 2

This site belongs to one of the country's best orthopedic hospitals. Bone, joint, and muscle-related diseases are its specialty, and it expertly provides patients with information about these conditions. Visit the patient education center and get happily lost in the fact sheets provided on the different types of arthritis and related conditions. I'm not exactly thrilled that there are links to pharmaceutical sponsors on the home page, but at least they are at the bottom of the page.

Johns Hopkins Arthritis Center
www.hopkins-arthritis.com

Source: 3
Navigation: 3
Interactivity: 2
Overall: 3

One of the country's best health care systems has produced an arthritis site that delivers. The information is well written and extremely credible. You'll read what the best minds in medicine have to say about the disease—enjoy it! The site also offers a long list of links to other resource centers. Don't leave without checking the message board or asking the expert a question.

Medical College of Wisconsin Arthritis and Rheumatic
    Diseases
www.healthlink.mcw.edu/arthritis

Source: 2
Navigation: 2
Interactivity: 1
Overall: 1

This site doesn't cover a lot of the arthritic conditions, but what it does cover, it does well. The site has information that's well resourced and, in many cases, drawn from equally credible websites dealing with arthritic diseases. Here you will be treated to the most recent news about arthritis and its treatment. This will not be the only place you will want to stop for information, but you might find a couple of articles that other sites haven't posted.

National Institute of Arthritis and Musculoskeletal and
  Skin Diseases
www.nih.gov/niams

Source: 3
Navigation: 1
Interactivity: 1
Overall: 1

Here you will find well-researched, easy-to-read patient-oriented brochures. Not all types of arthritis are covered, but enough of the major categories to satisfy most visitors. You can also order free information about arthritic conditions. The "News Releases" section, located on the home page, will keep you abreast of breaking news. Be prepared, however, to dig a little for the information.

Asthma

About.com on Asthma
www.asthma.about.com/mbody.htm

Source: 2
Navigation: 3
Interactivity: 2
Overall: 3

Sometimes you want to learn about the basics of a disease; other times you're looking for more advanced information. This site allows you to do both. In About's typical way, the site is designed for easy navigation and the content is written for all to understand. There are extensive options, ranging from learning about the latest asthma medications to viewing the anatomy of asthma and exactly what happens in the body. You will get the latest asthma news as well as learn which sports are asthma-friendly. If you want to talk to others who are living with asthma, join the chat room. This site won't leave you wanting much more.

American Academy of Allergy, Asthma
   and Immunology
www.aaaai.org

Source: 3
Navigation: 2
Interactivity: 1
Overall: 2

Here's another good place to get the basics on asthma, as well as the latest research updates. The information is easy to read, and the site is designed for easy access to information. Physician or patient, researcher or advocate, there's something here for everyone. You'll be glad you stopped here to learn more about asthma and how it might interact with your allergies.

American College of Allergy, Asthma & Immunology
   Online
www.allergy.mcg.edu

Source: 3
Navigation: 3
Interactivity: 3
Overall: 3

If you're looking for the best in asthma information, you must visit this site. Allergies are also covered, but the site's layout allows you to pick off the asthma information without having to go through the allergy information. This is a rock-solid website that you'll be happy to return to when looking for more asthma information.

American Lung Association
www.lungusa.org/asthma

Source: 3
Navigation: 3
Interactivity: 2
Overall: 3

What organization would have better asthma information for patients than the American Lung Association? The content on this site is current, well researched, and written at a level where both patient and doctor can understand. After navigating the site, you're left with one question: what doesn't it have? One of the special features is the "wall of remembrance" where survivors of those who've died from lung disease post memoriams for the deceased for everyone to read.

Asthma and Allergy Foundation of America
www.aafa.org

Source: 3
Navigation: 3
Interactivity: 2
Overall: 3

Once you log on, you'll want to stay for a long time. The information is just ready to be devoured; there's everything from facts and figures to FAQs to details on the latest research funded by the organization. If you speak Spanish, the information can be translated for you. Before finishing your reading, allow the resource links to take you to some of the most credible organizations in the world.

Canadian Lung Association
www.lung.ca/asthma

Source: 3
Navigation: 3
Interactivity: 2
Overall: 3

This site of the Canadian Lung Association is an excellent source to learn about asthma. While there may be differences in statistics and environmental relationships from one country to another, the basics of asthma are the same and this site does a commendable job of explaining it all to you. You can also access the "Guide to Prescription Drugs" and learn about the variety of asthma medications doctors frequently prescribe. You will leave this site well informed about asthma.

The Journal of the American Medical Association
   Asthma Information Center
www.ama-assn.org/special/asthma/treatmnt/
   treatmnt.htm

Source: 3
Navigation: 3
Interactivity: 1
Overall: 3

The Journal of the American Medical Association is one of the most respected medical journals in the world. This is the place where physicians want their research studies to be published because of its prestige and worldwide readership. It should come as no surprise that this site, which concentrates on asthma treatment—both clinical and medicinal—is backed by some of the latest and most validated of research. There is, however, a drawback: the site is written for a more advanced learner who already knows the basics of asthma. That said, there's a lot to learn here about asthma treatment. Try it, and you'll pick up a lot of useful information.

MayoClinic.com Allergy & Asthma Center
www.mayoclinic.com/home?id=3.1.1

Source: 3
Navigation: 2
Interactivity: 2
Overall: 2

The Mayo Clinic's Allergy and Asthma site does an excellent job of providing you with important asthma information without distractions. The language is simple and the style conducive to easy learning. Navigation is never a problem, as what you see is what you get. The links at the bottom of the page will send you to other Net resources that also provide good information. This is a great place to learn the no-nonsense basics.

National Asthma Campaign
www.asthma.org.uk

Source: 2
Navigation: 2
Interactivity: 1
Overall: 2

This is one of the largest asthma charities (foundations) in the United Kingdom. It provides easy-to-understand information about asthma and related issues. The site is constructed with the patient in mind, which makes navigating it quite easy. Children can also get into the act and enter the kids' zone to learn about their disease and ways to keep it under control. This is an all-around good site that's sure to answer many of your questions.

National Heart, Lung, and Blood Institute
www.nhlbi.nih.gov/health/public/lung/asthma/
   asth_fs.pdf

Source: 3
Navigation: 3
Interactivity: 1
Overall: 3

This site belongs to the National Heart, Lung, and Blood Institute, one of the premier research institutions in the world. This link is to its brochure on managing asthma. You can download the complete brochure and begin reading the basics that will carry you over to the more advanced topics. The booklet is full of interesting research and facts and figures that will educate you about asthma and ways of controlling it.

Attention Deficit Hyperactivity Disorder (ADHD)

American Academy of Pediatrics Practice Guidelines
   on ADHD
www.aap.org/policy/AC0002.html

Source: 3
Navigation: 1
Interactivity: 1
Overall: 1

This site serves one purpose: it gives you the practice guidelines of the American Academy of Pediatrics for diagnosing and evaluating children with suspected ADHD. There are no links, graphics, or any other basic website accessories. It's simply a document that states the positions of the country's foremost pediatric health professional organizations. Come to this site to learn how doctors might diagnose and evaluate your child for ADHD.

Children and Adults with Attention-Deficit/
    Hyperactivity Disorder
www.chadd.org

Source: 2
Navigation: 3
Interactivity: 2
Overall: 2

This well-rounded site will keep you up to speed on everything from the basics of ADHD to the legislative agenda concerning the disease in Washington, D.C. Besides providing the ABCs on ADHD, its biggest value is likely the fact sheet on debunking the myths surrounding many of the treatments. In an easy-to-follow sequence, it tells you what to look for and which rumored treatment strategies are more hoaxes than anything else. If you're looking for other ADHD websites and resources, this site will link you to a whole host of credible sources and allow you to enter a chat room to discuss ADHD with others having similar concerns. You'll leave this site better informed about ADHD.

Focus Adolescent Services
www.focusas.com/AttentionalDisorders.html

Source: 2
Navigation: 2
Interactivity: 2
Overall: 2

This website won't blow you away with fancy graphics or extraordinary links, but it does provide plenty of important information about the disease. It has a little something for most people, from holistic approaches to treating ADHD to a support group and resource center for parents. While I typically don't favor the selling of products on websites, the books that are offered could provide valuable information for families. If you are looking for one-stop shopping, this could be your site.

HealthAtoZ.com on ADHD
www.healthatoz.com/atoz/adhd/aindex.html

Source: 2
Navigation: 3
Interactivity: 3
Overall: 3

You can't go wrong looking for information on this site. It will link you to some of the most credible sources, and the editors frequently review the content to make sure it's current. You can post messages on the board or read those that others have written. You can also take a quiz to see if your child exhibits ADHD symptoms. The site offers a small but excellent list of sources that you can visit for more information. If you want reliable and succinct information on ADHD, this site won't let you down. If you take advantage of all of its content, you'll leave here a lot better informed than when you arrived.

Internet Mental Health
www.mentalhealth.com

Source: 3
Navigation: 3
Interactivity: 1
Overall: 2

I include this site for one reason: it draws information from the best sources on the Net. It allows you to access information in several formats including information booklets from professional or governmental organizations or magazine articles. If you want to surf the Web but don't have time to check out all of the sites on ADHD, this site is a good shortcut for getting reliable information quickly.

Kidsource Online on ADHD
www.kidsource.com

Source: 1
Navigation: 2
Interactivity: 1
Overall: 1

This site is designed differently from the others listed, so it will take some openness on your part to adjust to its presentation. Rather than organizing the site into different issues, such as the basics or treatment options, it provides a long queue of important information that is either linked to another website or opens up a page of text explaining the topic. The site is run by parents of children with ADHD, which gives it more insight into the social and family issues involved. If you're interested in reading about someone else's experiences, this would be a good place to start.

National Attention Deficit Disorder Association
www.add.org

Source: 2
Navigation: 2
Interactivity: 1
Overall: 2

You won't go wrong making this one of your first website visits when searching for ADHD info. It's quite an easy site to navigate because of its tidy organization, and all of the important links are right on the home page. Besides the ABCs on ADHD, the site has an excellent "Special Features" section that includes interviews with experts, people's personal stories, and a creative corner where people can express themselves. If you don't know what ADHD is or you want to share the experiences of others, you'll be pleased by what this site offers.

National Information Center for Children and Youth
    with Disabilities
www.nichcy.org

Source: 2
Navigation: 2
Interactivity: 1
Overall: 2

If you have some experience navigating websites, you'll need to put those skills to good use here. There is plenty of excellent information available, but the trick is to access it. Other sites go to great lengths to simplify your search for the basics, whereas this one makes you work a little harder. That said, once you do find the information, you can't help but be grateful. If you speak Spanish, "don't worry, be happy," there's information here for you also.

National Institute of Mental Health on Attention Deficit
    Hyperactivity Disorder
www.nimh.nih.gov/publicat/adhdmenu.cfm

Source: 3
Navigation: 3
Interactivity: 1
Overall: 3

If you don't know what ADHD is and you need the best information in the shortest amount of time, you should begin your search here. The National Institute of Mental Health delivers a large quantity of information about ADHD and its associated myths in plain talk. The information is also present in the coherent organizational style, which facilitates your search for a particular issue. You can learn the basics as well as the latest in research. There's something here for everyone, and you won't be distracted by a clutter of advertisements. Come here first, and you won't be disappointed.

Autoimmune Disorders

About.com on Autoimmune Disorders
www.rarediseases.about.com/cs/autoimmune

Source: 1
Navigation: 2
Interactivity: 2
Overall: 2

There aren't many autoimmune disorders that this site doesn't include, which makes it an important resource. While there is some original content on the site, its most valuable contribution is the long list of other Net resources to which it links. This is an excellent place to visit when you want to find other Internet sites and organizations that focus on a particular condition. If time permits, check out a chat on this topic.

American Autoimmune Related Diseases Association
www.aarda.org

Source: 3
Navigation: 3

Interactivity: 2
Overall: 3

If you visit this site first, you might not get to many others as the information is so accessible and satisfying. You can take your pick of facts about more than fifty-six autoimmune disorders, and once you've read all that's there, the links to other websites and Net resources will give you even more.

Arthritis Foundation
www.arthritis.org

Source: 3
Navigation: 3
Interactivity: 2
Overall: 2

While this is the site of the Arthritis Foundation, don't think that I've sent you here by accident. Many of the autoimmune disorders tend to overlap with the rheumatic diseases. Visit the Disease Center and look at the list of conditions. You will find some of the major autoimmune disorders also listed. Here you'll find good information at little navigation cost. If you find the disorder you're interested in, you're not likely to be disappointed.

Jewish Hospital HealthCare Services on Autoimmune
    Disorders
http://jhhs.client.web-health.com

Source: 2
Navigation: 1
Interactivity: 1
Overall: 1

Once you enter the website, just click on the "General Health" link, and you'll see a long list of topics that are covered. The autoimmune disorders section is quite extensive and written in a question-and-answer format that makes it easy to follow. This site won't blow you away with graphics or extensive links to other Net resources, but if you find your disease in the queue, you're in for a treat.

MEDLINEplus on Autoimmune Diseases
www.nlm.nih.gov/medlineplus/
autoimmunediseasesgeneral.html

Source: 3
Navigation: 3
Interactivity: 2
Overall: 2

MEDLINEplus is arguably the best database for medical information, covering a wide range of topics comprehensively and quickly. This site is no exception and is full of important information on a whole host of autoimmune disorders. You'll be satisfied with the quality of information and the other resources it links to. Stop here on your autoimmune information journey; you'll be happy you did.

National Institute of Allergy and Infectious Diseases on
Autoimmune Diseases
www.niaid.nih.gov/publications/autoimmune.htm

Source: 3
Navigation: 3
Interactivity: 1
Overall: 3

If you really want to learn about an autoimmune disorder, bookmark this website. The home page is quite busy, but it doesn't take away from the volume of information available to consumers. There is an important section on autoimmune disorders and, in what happens to be my favorite part, pictures and excellent explanations of the immune system and what goes wrong in the different autoimmune disorders. This site has enough solid information on it to keep you engrossed for hours, if not days.

National Organization for Rare Disorders
www.rarediseases.org

Source: 2
Navigation: 1
Interactivity: 2
Overall: 1

This website belongs to an organization comprising more than 140 not-for-profit voluntary health organizations dedicated to helping people who suffer from rare disorders and disabilities. Many of the autoimmune disorders fall under this category and can be found on this site. You will find links to other sites of rare disorders, and there's a link that explains what's available in the way of patient and family support. If no other site has the information you're looking for, there's a good chance it's here.

Office of Rare Diseases
http://rarediseases.info.nih.gov/ord

Source: 2
Navigation: 1
Interactivity: 2
Overall: 2

The Office of Rare Diseases provides information on more than six thousand rare diseases, some of which are autoimmune in nature. The information is less the ABCs of the disorders, more about research and current scientific news. If you're just starting your search, this is not the site to visit first. It will, however, be useful if you're interested in enrolling in or reading about clinical trials concerning your disease. You'll also find some good links for patient support groups and other information resources, as well as more advanced information.

Yahoo! Health on Autoimmune Disorders
http://dir.yahoo.com/Health/Diseases_and_Conditions/
    Autoimmune_Diseases/

Source: 1
Navigation: 3
Interactivity: 1
Overall: 1

Besides being a powerful search engine, Yahoo! provides some original content. It includes many of the autoimmune disorders in an easy-to-access list. You might want to try the site's long list of links to other Net resources. It's unclear who is actually providing the original content, and consumers would be better served with disclosure.

Back Pain

About.com on Orthopedics and Back Pain
www.orthopedics.about.com/blback.htm

Source: 3
Navigation: 3
Interactivity: 3
Overall: 3

This site is somewhat different from other sites reviewed because in addition to giving general information on some cases of back pain, it also gives you links to sites where you can find help. The difference between these links and other useful and related ones found on other sites is that this one has links to particular back pain situations instead of general ones.

Back Pain: University of Washington Orthopaedics and
   Sports Medicine
www.orthop.washington.edu/bonejoint/zlvzzzzz1_2.html

Source: 3
Navigation: 3
Interactivity: 1
Overall: 2

This page is part of a larger site sponsored by the University of Washington. It gives you just enough information to whet your appetite about back pain. It's an easy read and should answer your basic questions about the subject. For more detailed and specialist sites on back pain, pass this one up. If general information will suffice, this isn't a bad place to start.

Back Pain Answers
www.backpainanswers.com

Source: 1
Navigation: 3
Interactivity: 1
Overall: 1

This is a good site for those looking to learn more about back pain. It debunks many of the myths surrounding the subject and offers a simple and constructive discussion about diagnoses and treatments. There are advertisements, but only if you click on them will they interrupt your research.

BBC Online on Health and Fitness
www.bbc.co.uk/health/backchat

Source: 3
Navigation: 3
Interactivity: 1
Overall: 3

Here you'll find a nice "starter kit" approach to looking for answers regarding back pain. The information is simple yet effective, while the layout is spread out and not confused or cluttered. It's easy to find what you're looking for here. If you want more elaborate explanations or discussions, the site will disappoint. It's great if you just want to get your feet wet.

MEDLINEplus on Back Pain
www.nlm.nih.gov/medlineplus/backpain.html

Source: 3
Navigation: 3
Interactivity: 1
Overall: 3

This is one of the best sites for back pain information because of the varied resources employed. Like other MEDLINEplus topics, the discussion on back pain is beneficial to consumers because of the wide array of information presented. Renowned institutions from the National Institutes of Health to the Mayo Clinic have posted information for your use and convenience.

Spine-health.com
www.spine-health.com

Source: 3
Navigation: 3

Interactivity: 2
Overall: 3

If you have *any* questions about back pain, you will want to visit this comprehensive site. There's a wide array of topics to address your concerns. Navigation is a cinch, and it's a friendly site with plenty of content that has been thoughtfully put together.

Spine Universe
www.spineuniverse.com

Source: 3
Navigation: 3
Interactivity: 3
Overall: 3

There's a whole heap of information on this website, but don't let it overwhelm you. The site's clearly designed for people looking for real answers to back pain questions. Although the site's cluttered, it's easy to navigate and find what you're looking for. The listings are clear, so you can easily click on what interests you. The site features highly reputable contributors, is frequently updated, and includes many useful links. This is a must for questions concerning back pain.

National Institute of Neurological Disorders and Stroke
    Back Pain Information Page
www.ninds.nih.gov/health_and_medical/disorders/
    backpain_doc.htm

Source: 3
Navigation: 3
Interactivity: 1
Overall: 2

The information on this page is very brief but effective with regard to back pain. It is, however, best suited for the first-time back pain sufferer who hasn't really needed medical attention before. It doesn't go much into details on specific topics such as upper back pain, lower back pain, scoliosis, etc. Again, it's best for a consumer who thinks he or she is experiencing back pain and doesn't know why. Simple lifestyle changes are suggested that can help this type of person to alleviate back pain.

NeurologyChannel on Back Pain
www.neurologychannel.com/backpain

Source: 3
Navigation: 3
Interactivity: 3
Overall: 3

If you're experiencing back pain and scared to death because of it, this is a good site to visit. It's a very humanistic site, which after reading will leave you feeling that you're not alone. Also, it lets you know that you don't have to wave the white flag because of the discomfort you are experiencing. Emphasis is placed on short-term back pain, although more severe symptoms aren't ignored.

Yahoo! Health on Nonspecific Back Pain
http://health.yahoo.com/health/Diseases_And_
    Conditions/Disease_Feed_Data/nonspecific_
    back_pain

Source: 3
Navigation: 3
Interactivity: 3
Overall: 3

Yes, the URL is long, but once you're past that, you're golden. The sites selected for review, in general, are designed to be nonspecific. They're meant for both the consumer who knows what the problem is and the one who doesn't. You can read up on definitions of back pain to see if that's really the source of your discomfort. Also, information on causes and symptoms as well as signs to watch for and tests to take can be clicked on, depending on your interests. It's really a site where the consumer has control, thus eliminating excess time and unwanted information.

Cancer

American Cancer Society
www.cancer.org

Source: 3
Navigation: 3
Interactivity: 3
Overall: 3

The ACS has a long history of providing quality cancer information, and this site is bursting at the seams with it. This is one of the Net's best places to begin and in some cases end your search for cancer information. Not only is it easy to navigate, it contains information in Spanish as well. The site also has excellent interactive options, such as an online community of cancer survivors. You can also try the "Cancer Profiler," an interactive tool that enables cancer patients and their physicians to make better-informed treatment decisions using information from evidence-based, peer-reviewed medical literature. If every site were as thorough and well resourced as this one, there would be no need for this book.

cancerfacts.com
www.cancerfacts.com

Source: 1
Navigation: 2
Interactivity: 2
Overall: 2

This site makes use of cutting-edge technology that allows you to input personal information about your health, preferences, and cancer and gives you a report on possible treatment options. There is a very clear warning that the information provided is by no means a substitute for a physician, but rather information that might stimulate conversation with your doctor. It's clear and easy to read, and it takes no more than fifteen to twenty minutes to answer the questions and read the resulting report. There are also links to other studies that you can read to get a better understanding of the latest and greatest treatment options. This isn't a site to use if you've just been diagnosed with cancer and you want to learn more about it. Instead, this is a site for those who already know something about their cancer and want to focus on treatment options.

CancerGuide
www.cancerguide.org

Source: N/A
Navigation: N/A
Interactivity: N/A
Overall: 2

This is a site that directs you to other sources on the Internet. If you want specific information and fact sheets, this isn't your site. However, if you want to investigate several types of cancer or issues related to cancer, this site provides an enormous list of links.

CancerLinks
www.cancerlinks.com

Source: N/A
Navigation: N/A
Interactivity: N/A
Overall: 1

Although this site does not post original content, it efficiently directs you to a vast amount of worthwhile cancer-specific information. Here you will find one of the most comprehensive, best-organized group of cancer links you'll ever see. You will be able to scan the Internet in the corners of the globe with just a few clicks. One of the great links is a cancer support link that addresses the issues surrounding cancer care, such as nutrition, exercise, fatigue, and pain control. If you want one site that can lead you to hundreds of others, this should be your first stop.

CancerNet
www.cancernet.nci.nih.gov

Source: 3
Navigation: 3
Interactivity: 2
Overall: 3

This is the site of the powerful National Cancer Institute, full of the world's leading research compiled from scientists and databases. That said, it's made specifically for consumers, providing easy-to-read content and constructed so it's easy to navigate. The information is updated frequently, and the resources and support the site provides are also first rate. Here you can also learn about entering a clinical trial for the latest treatment. This site is a must for anyone diagnosed with cancer or looking for information for a loved one.

Cancer Research Foundation of America
www.crfa.org

Source: 3
Navigation: 2
Interactivity: 1
Overall: 2

Although I'm on the board of directors of this organization, the following praise is entirely unbiased and well deserved. This site is dedicated to preventing cancer and providing funds to cancer researchers. The information is credible, easy to read, and presented in both English and Spanish. The site nicely breaks down the major cancers between men and women, then looks at your risk for each based on your age. There's a special section called "Hope Street Kids" that provides extensive information about childhood cancers. Not many organizations or websites are devoted to prevention. This site carries that distinction as a badge of honor and delivers on its promise.

CancerSource.com
www.cancersource.com

Source: 2
Navigation: 1
Interactivity: 3
Overall: 2

This site has an excellent advisory board and a vast range of material on different types of cancers. While this is a good site to visit once you have been diagnosed with cancer, it can be a little more cumbersome than others to navigate. However, what the site lacks in other areas, it more than makes up for in the interactivity department. You can join a chat room, read or post to a message board, join a mailing list, or participate in a support group. If interaction is your driving force, look no further.

Harvard Center for Cancer Prevention
www.hsph.harvard.edu/cancer

Source: 3
Navigation: 3
Interactivity: 2
Overall: 3

This site is dedicated to preventing cancer and providing important information that can help you do just that! The site is extremely well organized and a cinch to navigate. The links are laid out very simply, and there's no need to dig for the information because it's all there so clearly. There's an excellent new interactive feature: how to predict your cancer risk. It puts you through a series of questions and answers and at the end estimates your cancer risk for the twelve leading cancers and gives you tips for prevention. This is an important website because it addresses cancer when it's most curable—before it occurs.

OncoLink
www.oncolink.upenn.edu

Source: 3
Navigation: 3
Interactivity: 2
Overall: 3

This extremely credible academic site has won several big Internet awards. The information provided is well documented and frequently updated. The site's clear organization and easy navigation help consumers take advantage of its many offerings, including online support groups in which you can read other people's stories or, if you wish, tell your own. There are so many offerings at this site, you can spend hours and hours there and still feel that you could spend more.

Oncology.com
www.oncology.com

Source: 3
Navigation: 3
Interactivity: 3
Overall: 3

This site provides extensive information on most cancers as well as a lot of resources dedicated to the latest in cancer news. One of this site's strengths is its interactive tools. You can do everything from locating hospitals and doctors to finding a clinical trial in which you can enroll to test new treatments. One of the special features could be its most important: "cancer buddy" online chat. This site is easy to navigate and full of interesting links that address the cancer experience from a global perspective. With its well-respected editorial board and well-researched information, this site must be one of your primary information-gathering stops on the Internet.

Breast Cancer

American Breast Cancer Foundation
www.abcf.org

Source: 2
Navigation: 3
Interactivity: 1
Overall: 2

This foundation's mission is to help lead the fight for a breast cancer cure, encourage early detection, and support women and their families dealing with breast cancer. Its website is a reflection of this mission. The information is written in a straightforward manner and the site is user-friendly, allowing you to access the desired information without hassle. The links to support groups, advocacy groups, and other Net resources are quite extensive. I really like the mammogram reminder feature, which sends you an e-mail to let you know when it's time to have your next mammogram. This site is simple but informative.

American Cancer Society on Breast Cancer
www3.cancer.org/cancerinfo/load_cont.asp?ct=5&
    language=English

Source: 3
Navigation: 3
Interactivity: 1
Overall: 2

You've come to the right place to get the ABCs on breast cancer. But while you're here, you can also take a quiz that tests your knowledge or read a guide to performing a breast self-exam. The links at the bottom of the page are excellent, and if you click on them, you'll find yourself on some of the best breast cancer sites. Make this a must-stop on the breast cancer information journey.

BreastCancer.Net
www.breastcancer.net

Source: 2
Navigation: 2
Interactivity: 1
Overall: 1

This site is the one to visit if you want the latest in breast cancer news, whether treatment or diagnosis. You can still get the basics on this site, and the good news is that it draws much of its information from other credible sites and organizations such as the American Cancer Society. The links to other resources are an excellent way to expand your search if what you find here isn't enough.

Cancerlinks on Breast Cancer
www.cancerlinks.org/breast.html

Source: N/A
Navigation: N/A
Interactivity: N/A
Overall: 1

This site has one major purpose: to connect you to an extensive array of sources on the Internet that can provide you with breast cancer information. There are at least sixteen different languages to choose from, and the site organizes the links into several categories. Whether you are looking for emotional support or answers to questions on hormone replacement therapy, this site will quickly direct you to other sources that can provide the information. All in all, this is a great doorway to breast cancer information on the Net.

Mayo Clinic
www.mayoclinic.com/home?id=SP3.1.5.6

Source: 3
Navigation: 3
Interactivity: 1
Overall: 2

The Mayo Clinic, one of the world's most respected medical institutions, has made finding cancer information easy for you on this site. It's divided into the different stages of cancer: understanding, preventing, treating, and living with the disease. You can't help but leave this site much better informed about the different aspects of cancer and its many controversies.

National Alliance of Breast Cancer Organizations
www.nabco.org

Source: 3
Navigation: 3
Interactivity: 3
Overall: 3

The National Alliance of Breast Cancer Organizations is a non-profit information and education resource on breast cancer that has a network of more than four hundred member organizations nationwide. This site has information for everyone, medical professionals and patients alike. Material on this site has been scientifically reviewed. The site is easy to navigate, and some of the interactive tools include transcripts of past online chats. This is a site you must visit when searching for breast cancer information.

Oncology.com
www.oncology.com

Source: 3
Navigation: 3
Interactivity: 3
Overall: 3

You can stay on this site for hours on end, trying to digest all of the excellent information. It's written for a layperson, and the site organization is such that navigation is a cinch. You will learn about all aspects of breast cancer and have the opportunity to chat online with someone facing a similar challenge.

This is a great place to do your one-stop breast cancer information shopping.

Oncologychannel.com on Breast Cancer
www.oncologychannel.com/breastcancer

Source: 3
Navigation: 3
Interactivity: 3
Overall: 3

Click for click, one of the best breast cancer information sites on the Net. The information seems endless, and it's written in a way that makes it easy to read and digest. There are several features that make it stand out, such as its chemotherapy forum, where you can ask about the side effects of chemotherapy, and the "Hopelink" link, which helps you find clinical trials to participate in. This site could be your first and only stop when looking for breast cancer info.

Susan G. Komen Breast Cancer Foundation
www.komen.org

Source: 2
Navigation: 3
Interactivity: 2
Overall: 2

This is one of the most visible breast cancer foundations in the United States. It has raised more than $100 million for cancer research, education, and support. This site allows you to access the excellent information the foundation has prepared for breast cancer patients and their families. You can read about the basics of breast cancer and the latest headline breast cancer news. Don't leave this site off your breast cancer information tour.

Colon Cancer

American Cancer Society on Colon Cancer
www3.cancer.org/cancerinfo/load_cont.asp?ct=1&
    language=English

Source: 3
Navigation: 3
Interactivity: 3
Overall: 3

The American Cancer Society, one of the largest and most respected cancer organizations in the world, has built a site that
stands head and shoulders above most others. It has easy-to-
read information that explains a variety of topics from prevention and risk factors to the latest treatments available. The
interactive tools are also first-rate, as you can tune in to a webcast on colon cancer or calculate your risk of getting this type
of cancer. This site has something for everyone, and you should
use it for all it's worth—a lot.

American College of Gastroenterology
www.acg.gi.org/acg-dev/patientinfo/frame_
    coloncancer.html

Source: 3
Navigation: 3
Interactivity: 1
Overall: 2

Something we all look for when searching for information
about a dangerous illness is a ray of hope that all will be fine.
Obviously that depends on the condition, but something else
that can make the information easier to digest is a website that's
well designed, on which information is easy to access, rather

than requiring you to perform an arduous search. Well, this site delivers and then some. You will be informed about screening exams, prevention tips, and fact sheets. Sit back and relax and let the links work for you.

American Gastroenterological Association
www.gastro.org/public/cc_screening.html

Source: 2
Navigation: 3
Interactivity: 2
Overall: 2

The public section of this website has all of the information neatly stored and ready to be absorbed. This prestigious association does an excellent job of breaking down the subject of colon cancer into many related issues and presenting them in a format that makes finding the information effortless. Read the basics, then check out the message boards to hear what other colon cancer patients and doctors have to say. If you have extra time, check out other GI problems—why not kill two birds with one stone?

Cancer Care on Colon Cancer
www.cancercare.org/campaigns/colon1.htm

Source: 2
Navigation: 3
Interactivity: 3
Overall: 2

If you or a loved one has been diagnosed with colon cancer, this website is as good as any other to find credible information and share the experience of others. You can read the fact sheets about diagnosis and prevention, then click on a link to order a free online publication. While you're here and have some free time, listen to one of the cancer care teleconferences online. You never know what you might learn from the leading experts who participate in them!

Cancerlinks on Colon Cancer
www.cancerlinks.org/colon.html

Source: N/A
Navigation: N/A
Interactivity: N/A
Overall: 1

If you want the one place on the Internet that has the most colon cancer links, this is it. The purpose of this site is simply to link you to other resources on the Net that cover a wide range of colon cancer–related issues from clinical trials you can join to safety tips when traveling on airplanes. This site is an important gateway that opens up the World Wide Web of colon cancer information.

National Cancer Institute: CancerNet on Colon Cancer
www.cancernet.nci.nih.gov/Cancer_Types/Colon_And_
    Rectal_Cancer.shtml

Source: 3
Navigation: 3
Interactivity: 2
Overall: 3

The National Cancer Institute is one of the world's foremost cancer research centers, and this site helps distinguish it as one of the most important Net sources for colon cancer information. Navigating the website is extremely easy, and you'll be as amazed as I was at how thorough and well written it is. There are pages for support and links to other resources. If you need colon cancer information, you'll hit pay dirt on this site.

National Colorectal Cancer Research Alliance
www.nccra.org

Source: 1
Navigation: 3
Interactivity: 1
Overall: 1

The *Today* show's Katie Couric and the Entertainment Industry Foundation have cofounded this alliance with the support of several corporations to get the word out about colorectal cancer, particularly how important screening can be in saving lives. The information is easy to read, and the site is a navigation breeze. Once you've read what the site has to offer, link to other sites that can provide answers to your remaining questions. Sometimes a big name and big money can be put to use for the public good.

OncoLink on Colon Cancer
www.oncolink.upenn.edu/disease/colorectal

Source: 3
Navigation: 3
Interactivity: 2
Overall: 3

This site belongs to the University of Pennsylvania Cancer Center, and it is worthy of its Ivy League credential. The information is of excellent quality and written to make difficult concepts easy to understand. There's a plethora of information that will get you up to speed in no time. As a bonus, you can easily

click on links to information on other cancers and quickly discover more content that's equally noteworthy.

Oncology.com on Colorectal Cancer
www.oncology.com

Source: 3
Navigation: 3
Interactivity: 3
Overall: 3

When I'm looking for cancer information, this is one of the first
sites I check. It has an excellent medical advisory board, and
the site is dedicated to getting the information right without
taking shortcuts. The site is so good I don't know where to
start. The information is extensive, and the site is extremely
well organized. The interactive tools are some of the best, and
the resource links provide even more information. You would
be remiss to look for colon cancer information without stopping here.

Oncologychannel.com on Colorectal Cancer
www.oncologychannel.com/coloncancer

Source: 3
Navigation: 3
Interactivity: 3
Overall: 3

This site is one of the best places to do your one-stop colon cancer information shopping. It has extensive information, and the
site is organized for simple navigation. If you have the guts to
do it, take a look inside the abdomen and see what the colon
looks like. Sign up for a chat, find an oncologist near you, or
check out the many links to other sites. Once you're here, you
may feel that there's no reason to go anywhere else.

Lung Cancer

American Cancer Society on Lung Cancer
www3.cancer.org/cancerinfo/load_cont.asp?ct=26&
   language=English

Source: 3
Navigation: 3
Interactivity: 1
Overall: 3

The American Cancer Society is one of the greatest cancer organizations in the world. Its site is completely patient-friendly,
covering a wide range of lung cancer–related issues in language and format that are easy to understand. If you only speak
Spanish, *no te preocupes*—there are content pages here for you
also. Credible information, easy navigation, well-written fact
sheets—your answers are here.

American Lung Association
www.lungusa.org/diseases/lungcanc.html

Source: 3
Navigation: 3
Interactivity: 1
Overall: 2

This site offers you the basics about lung cancer. There isn't
much fanfare, and there aren't any big interactive tools such as
chats or message boards. This is a site to visit when you want
just the facts in a no-hassle manner. At the bottom of the page,
you're also directed to a few other resources that can provide
valuable information. This is not likely to be your only stop for
lung cancer information, but it could be helpful along the way.

CancerLinks on Lung Cancer
www.cancerlinks.org/lung.html

Source: N/A
Navigation: N/A
Interactivity: N/A
Overall: 1

This site has one goal: to provide you with the most lung cancer links on the Net. It can direct you in several different languages, and it covers a wide range of issues related to lung cancer. If you're at a loss as to where to search for more lung cancer–related sites, this site is the answer.

Cancer Research Foundation of America
www.crfa.org

Source: 2
Navigation: 2
Interactivity: 2
Overall: 2

This organization is all about prevention, and while its content conveys this message, you'll still get all the basics about lung cancer. The way the site is designed, you have to navigate a bit before arriving at the lung cancer information, but it's well worth the extra clicks. The information is easy to read and well researched. You know you're reading credible information when you peruse the pages on this site.

Lungcancer.org
www.lungcancer.org

Source: 2
Navigation: 3

Interactivity: 3
Overall: 2

This site is well designed, and the information is easy to follow. There are different entry points for patients and caregivers, health professionals, and media. You can learn about lung cancer from A to Z on this site and, once you've conquered the basics, read recent lung cancer headlines or reports from recent meetings. The interactive tools are excellent, allowing you to read the personal accounts of those with similar stories or ask an expert a question. If you visit this site, plan to spend a fair amount of time to absorb all that's offered.

MayoClinic.com on Lung Cancer
www.mayoclinic.com/home?id=DS00038

Source: 3
Navigation: 3
Interactivity: 1
Overall: 2

The Mayo Clinic is one of those venerable organizations that just breathes credibility. The information on these pages is patient-friendly, and the site is easy to navigate. Your basic questions will be answered, as will your concerns about coping with lung cancer. The list of links to additional resources isn't lengthy, but the sites it does refer to are of the highest caliber. You'll leave this site well informed about the effects of this potentially devastating disease.

Medem
www.medem.com

Source: 3
Navigation: 3

Interactivity: 1
Overall: 3

Medem is a library of information that has been provided and approved by the nation's leading medical societies. The information is easy to read, extremely credible, and organized in a way that makes navigating easy. Beyond the facts, there are articles that deal with more specific issues and may be of interest to you. Try just browsing; you never know what pearl of wisdom you'll come across.

National Cancer Institute: CancerNet on Lung Cancer
www.cancernet.nci.nih.gov/cancer_types/lung_cancer.
   shtml

Source: 3
Navigation: 3
Interactivity: 2
Overall: 3

The country's leading cancer research institution delivers a site that lets patients and their families understand lung cancer and its related issues. You'll read information from how lung cancer is diagnosed to what some of the most recent treatment regimens are being used to combat it. You can also find out if there's a clinical trial you might qualify to participate in or check a few of the many links the site has to other Net sources—though you might not need to visit them after navigating this site!

Oncology.com
www.oncology.com

Source: 3
Navigation: 3

Interactivity: 3
Overall: 3

This is one of the best lung cancer information sites on the Net. The design is extremely friendly and easy to use, and your entry point is based on your experience or desired information. The content is thorough, thoughtful, and frequently reviewed for accuracy. You can also use important interactive tools such as the "cancer buddy" chat, which allows you to talk with someone else with a similar problem. This is what a website that intends to inform the public should look like.

Oncologychannel.com on Lung Cancer
www.oncologychannel.com/lungcancer

Source: 2
Navigation: 3
Interactivity: 3
Overall: 3

This is one of the one-stop shopping sites where you can do everything without needing to type in another URL. The site is designed to make your search as effortless and convenient as possible. It's easy to find what you're looking for, as everything is clearly laid out. You can chat with other patients or experts or ask the doctor a question. Even if this is your first stop for information, it might well be your last.

Ovarian Cancer

CancerGuide
www.cancerguide.org

Source: N/A
Navigation: N/A

Interactivity: N/A
Overall: 2

This site is a must for the novice online researcher. It contains valuable information on conducting a search, source reliability, and practical tips about interpreting scientific data. The tone is no-nonsense and straightforward and makes navigating the somewhat cluttered site worthwhile.

Cancer 411
www.411cancer.com

Source: 1
Navigation: 3
Interactivity: 1
Overall: 2

If you want the 411 on clinical trials and current developments in cancer treatment, this is a good place to start. The information here is very comprehensive. Don't end your search here, however, as this site presents all new treatment options, some of which may be of questionable benefit.

CyberMedTrials.org
www.cybermedtrials.com

Source: 3
Navigation: 2
Interactivity: 2
Overall: 2

Ovarian cancer patients looking for information on the latest cancer treatments can find it on this site. It contains an easy-to-read, searchable database of clinical trials organized by state. It also contains a great database of support groups, a chemotherapy side effects manual, a medical dictionary, and a "General Information" section.

The Gilda Radner Familial Ovarian Cancer Registry
www.ovariancancer.com/grwp.html

Source: 2
Navigation: 2
Interactivity: 1
Overall: 2

This site is for those who have relatives with ovarian cancer and are worried about their risk of getting the disease. It offers a toll-free help line, educational materials, and support for women with a high risk of ovarian cancer.

Johns Hopkins Ovarian Cancer
www.ovariancancer.jhmi.edu

Source: 3
Navigation: 3
Interactivity: 1
Overall: 2

This is a great resource not only for information on ovarian cancer but also for moral support. The site contains inspirational stories from ovarian cancer patients in their own words.

National Ovarian Cancer Association Ovarian Cancer
    Research Notebook
www.slip.net/~mcdavis/ovarian.html

Source: 2
Navigation: 2
Interactivity: 3
Overall: 2

This is a comprehensive site of organized treatment for advanced ovarian cancer with summaries of cutting-edge research that are easily accessible by patients and professionals alike.

National Ovarian Cancer Coalition
www.ovarian.org

Source: 3
Navigation: 3
Interactivity: 1
Overall: 3

If you or someone you love has been diagnosed with ovarian cancer and you're looking for comprehensive information about the disease, this is the site to begin your search. Initially developed by a forty-seven-year-old woman with stage III ovarian cancer, the site contains thousands of patient-friendly resources containing complete and accurate information, including medical consultation through its "Ask the Experts" section, information on clinical trials, and a national database of gynecologic oncologists.

OncoLink on Ovarian Cancer
www.oncolink.upenn.edu/specialty/gyn_onc/ovarian

Source: 3
Navigation: 3
Interactivity: 2
Overall: 3

This site contains comprehensive, up-to-date information on cancer, cancer treatment, and current research. It is organized to provide information at the level you're most comfortable with, ranging from basic, introductory information to advanced, in-depth information. If you're interested in learning about any type of cancer, this is the site for you.

Ovarian Cancer National Alliance
www.ovariancancer.org

Source: 2
Navigation: 3
Interactivity: 2
Overall: 2

This is a well-organized site with information geared toward the newly diagnosed, friends and family, survivors, and those interested in general information on cancer.

Quackwatch
www.quackwatch.com

Source: 2
Navigation: 2
Interactivity: 1
Overall: 2

This site is an excellent resource for any patient considering unconventional therapy. Dr. Steven Barrett has developed a feature section specifically for cancer patients whose desperation may cause them to pursue dubious treatments. If you want to make intelligent choices about treatment, the section "Questionable Cancer Treatments" is a must-read.

Prostate Cancer

American Cancer Society on Prostate Cancer
www3.cancer.org/cancerinfo/load_cont.asp?ct=36&
    language=English

Source: 3
Navigation: 3

Interactivity: 2
Overall: 3

This is one of the most trusted cancer organizations in the world. Its information is easy to read and draws on an extremely large database of statistics and research. When I'm looking for cancer information, this is a must-read for me. You can also use the site's interactive tools, such as the cancer profiler, which combines three decision tools to help you evaluate which treatment options are best for you. Don't leave without checking its links to other cancer sources.

American Foundation for Urologic Disease on Prostate
    Cancer
www.afud.org/conditions/pc.html

Source: 2
Navigation: 3
Interactivity: 1
Overall: 1

Get the basics of prostate cancer from an important foundation that deals with an array of urologic diseases of which prostate cancer is one of the most important. This site keeps it simple, and its design is uncomplicated. Find out the ABCs of prostate cancer, and if you're feeling knowledgeable about the disease put your brain to the test with the prostate cancer quiz.

Brady Urological Institute at Johns Hopkins University
http://prostate.urol.jhu.edu/diseases/prostate/prostate.
    html#button3

Source: 2
Navigation: 2
Interactivity: 1
Overall: 1

This site is most concerned with giving you credible information in as easy accessible a manner as possible. There aren't any interactive tools and there are no real links to external Net resources, but the information is comprehensive and well presented. This should not be your only stop for information, but it's one that you can trust.

MayoClinic.com on Prostate Cancer
www.mayoclinic.com/home?id=DS00043

Source: 3
Navigation: 3
Interactivity: 1
Overall: 2

What are the symptoms of prostate cancer, and when should you go to your doctor to make sure all is well? These questions and others are answered by this information-loaded site, which delivers some of the best prostate cancer content on the Net. Before you go on to other sites, make sure you have the basics down; visiting this site will help you do so.

National Cancer Institute: CancerNet on Prostate Cancer
cancernet.nci.nih.gov/Cancer_Types/Prostate_Cancer.
  shtml

Source: 3
Navigation: 3
Interactivity: 2
Overall: 3

This site of the prestigious National Cancer Institute offers practically everything you would ever want to know on prostate cancer. If it doesn't, using the links to other sources will finish the job. You'll get not only the basics but the latest in prostate cancer research and current treatment recommendations. The site also has an important link for support groups and resources. Stopping here could be one of the most important stops you make when looking for prostate cancer information on the Net.

Oncolink on Prostate Cancer
http://cancer.med.upenn.edu/disease/prostate

Source: 3
Navigation: 3
Interactivity: 2
Overall: 3

This is one of those sites where once you start to find information, you can't help but look for more. The site is well organized and gives consumers a chance to access information with little effort. Here you can learn the basics of prostate cancer as well as its various treatments. Your search will also turn up links to support groups and information about how to cope with prostate cancer and its related issues. If you have limited time to search for information, this site can deliver quality information in a hurry.

Oncology.com on Prostate Cancer
www.oncology.com

Source: 2
Navigation: 3
Interactivity: 3
Overall: 3

This site takes the different aspects of prostate cancer and wraps them up neatly so that users can digest information quickly and with minimal effort. Learn about a variety of issues, including symptoms, treatment, and statistics. The interactive part of the site is excellent, allowing chats between cancer patients and helping patients figure out their risk for cancer. Don't be surprised if this site answers all of your prostate-related questions.

Oncologychannel.com on Prostate Cancer
www.oncologychannel.com/prostatecancer

Source: 2
Navigation: 3
Interactivity: 3
Overall: 3

What more can you ask for in a website on prostate cancer than what is here? You'll find in-depth yet easy-to-read information that takes you through the basics of prostate cancer and suggests questions you might ask your doctor. The interactive tools are excellent, allowing you to ask a doctor questions, find an oncologist (cancer doctor) near you, or participate in a live chat. This well-rounded site could possibly answer all of your prostate cancer questions.

Prostate Cancer Research Foundation of Canada
www.prostatecancer.on.ca

Source: 2
Navigation: 3
Interactivity: 1
Overall: 2

This site belongs to Canada's leading national organization devoted to eliminating prostate cancer. It provides information on prostate cancer in its "Quick Facts" link. Learn everything from what the prostate does in the body to the symptoms of prostate cancer. Read stories of courage and learn how to cope when you or a loved one has the disease. This site isn't just for patients but for anyone wanting to learn more about this very treatable disease.

> University of Michigan Urologic Oncology Program on Prostate Cancer
> www.cancer.med.umich.edu/prostcan/prostcan.html
>
> *Source: 2*
> *Navigation: 2*
> *Interactivity: 1*
> *Overall: 2*

This site, which belongs to the University of Michigan Comprehensive Cancer Center, channels the center's vast resources so that you can learn about one of the most common cancers in men. As with most academic sites, the information is quite credible, and the site is organized to make navigation simple. You can find out about ongoing clinical trials for prostate cancer patients and take advantage of the excellent links that send you to other sources of information.

Children's Health, General

> About.com on Pediatrics
> www.pediatrics.about.com/health/pediatrics/mbody.htm?IAM=vpn000586_1
>
> *Source: 1*
> *Navigation: 1*
> *Interactivity: 2*
> *Overall: 1*

Most of the content on this site is not original content from About.com, but rather content from other sites gathered in one spot for the visitor. It's hard to tell what's original and what's not—but the bottom line is that it's an accumulation of a lot of health information, so it's worth checking out—just be careful about the source and double-check what you learn against material from other sources.

CBS HealthWatch on Parenting
www.cbshealthwatch.medscape.com/parentingcenter

Source: 3
Navigation: 3
Interactivity: 2
Overall: 2

An excellent consumer health site owned by Medscape, which is a leading medical website for physicians. Most of the content is vetted by medical experts. It covers every major health condition and is updated frequently. It provides feature articles for the newly diagnosed as well as more knowledgeable patients and caregivers, current news, FAQs, an "ask the expert" option, community features, a wealth of resources and searches through the library, related links, and much more. This site should act as a great starting point to learn more about child health and where to go for more detailed information.

Centers for Disease Control and Prevention: The ABC's
of Safe and Healthy Child Care
www.cdc.gov/ncidod/hip/abc/abc.htm

Source: 3
Navigation: 3
Interactivity: 1
Overall: 3

You can't get much more credible than the CDC. This online manual is a solid guide to health and safety issues for children, although it was obviously not originally intended for online use, as there are no other website resource addresses or links. Additionally, one of the great things about the Net is how easy it is to update and revise material, but the CDC has not taken advantage of that capability. As of this writing, much of the content has not been updated or revised in the past few years, and many items on the Fact Sheet and Table of Contents are dated January 1997. Don't be alarmed, though—it's all still relevant and a good resource for health and safety.

FDA Kids
www.fda.gov/oc/opacom/kids

Source: 3
Navigation: 3
Interactivity: 1
Overall: 3

Credibility is never in question with the Food and Drug Administration, and neither is navigation on this somewhat simple and aesthetically appealing website for kids. This site focuses on foods, vaccines, poisons, animals, medicine, and parenting. While it's not purely a site on child health, it's very good at covering these major health topics and is an excellent resource for pediatric nutrition and drug information.

healthfinder kids
www.healthfinder.gov/kids

Source: 3
Navigation: 1
Interactivity: 1
Overall: 3

The Office of Disease Prevention and Health Promotion, U.S. Department of Health and Human Services, created http://www.healthfinder.gov in 1997. The kids' section featured here was created in 2000. This is a good place to find all related links created by the U.S. government, and more. Though you would hope that anything offered by the U.S. Department of Health and Human Services would be highly credible, remember that you will be surfing from this site to other child health websites, sometimes not created by the U.S. government. Nevertheless, it's user-friendly, fun for kids, and not too overwhelming. Some information on the parent website, www.healthfinder.gov, is provided in Spanish.

> iVillage.com on Child Health
> www.ivillage.com/topics/family/health
>
> *Source: 2*
> *Navigation: 1*
> *Interactivity: 2*
> *Overall: 1*

This site contains so much information and places to communicate with others, it can be overwhelming and confusing; in fact, at times I wondered what website I was on. Overall, however, it is a solid place to search for information on your child's health—and chat with other caregivers on topics of child care.

> Keep Kids Healthy
> www.keepkidshealthy.com
>
> *Source: 2*
> *Navigation: 1*
> *Interactivity: 2*
> *Overall: 1*

Navigating through this site is painfully slow, even with a cable modem! Banner ads and e-commerce on the home page and throughout the website, along with redundant information, make using this site rather difficult. However, many of the features are (usually) worth the wait—fun/different tools, as well as good resources and health information to help parents improve their children's health and safety. And a free customized newsletter for your child based on age, with appropriate information on nutrition, growth, development, safety, vaccines, and more, is available.

KidsGrowth.com
www.kidsgrowth.com
Or go directly to KidsGrowth Child Health at
www.kidsgrowth.com/index2.cfm

Source: 2
Navigation: 3
Interactivity: 2
Overall: 2

A website that offers much more than just basic health information. The site offers articles on parenting and behavior; information on child development categorized by age group, childhood conditions, major growth milestones, and parenting resources; parenting tips; information on product recalls; reviews of children's books; an "ask the expert" option; and even a free KidsGrowth weekly e-mail newsletter. Here you'll find a plethora of resources and options for educating yourself on your child's health. Fairly clearly laid out and largely user-friendly, this website should be on your list of places to visit when researching children's health issues.

KidsHealth
www.kidshealth.org

Source: 3
Navigation: 3
Interactivity: 1
Overall: 3

Simply put, I liked this site from the start. Created for kids and parents by Nemours Foundation, a nonprofit organization devoted to children's health. KidsHealth.org provides up-to-date information about growth, food and fitness, childhood infections, immunizations, lab tests, medical conditions, and the latest treatments. This site successfully educates three very different audiences on the topic of childhood health; using different colors, language, and tools, the site effectively communicates the messages. A top-notch site.

Patient Education Program
www.cincinnatichildrens.org/family/pep

Source: 3
Navigation: 3
Interactivity: 1
Overall: 3

From the Children's Hospital Medical Center of Cincinnati, this is a site that contains a series of articles that help children and their families understand basic medical conditions, medications, tests, and procedures. Included are guides to home care and wellness. The site is well written and organized, with drop-down menus throughout the site that make seeking information easy and allow the user to see all options available at all times. This is a highly credible and useful website on which to research your child's health.

Chiropractic

Chiropractors
www.allsands.com/money/career/chiropractors_xok_
    gn.htm

Source: 1
Navigation: 3
Interactivity: 1
Overall: 1

This is an informative site that explains what a chiropractor is
and does. Its content is objective, though its subject matter remains a hot-button issue. After reading this, you will have an
insight into the supply and demand out there for chiropractors
and the reasons. What you won't be able to do after reading
this, however, is decide whether or not chiropractic is for you.

McLaughlin Chiropractic Center: The Chiropractic
    Handbook
www.mclaughlinchiropractic.com/handbook/Main_
    Handbook.htm

Source: 3
Navigation: 3
Interactivity: 1
Overall: 2

If you're considering chiropractic and you don't have a clue
about its merits, this is a good site for you. It answers many of
the questions associated with chiropractic that you might have
about the practice and its practitioners. Be forewarned, however, that chiropractic's merits are still under discussion in the
medical world—and that on this site an avowed adherent is discussing its merits.

Paralumun New Age Womens Village on Chiropractors
www.paralumun.com/chiropractors.htm

Source: 1
Navigation: 3
Interactivity: 1
Overall: 1

This site gives a brief history of chiropractic and how its use has increased over the years. It talks briefly about how chiropractors diagnose and treat patients. It's neither a site "for" nor a site "against" chiropractic.

Chronic Fatigue Syndrome

About.com on Chronic Fatigue Syndrome/Fibromyalgia
www.chronicfatigue.about.com/health/chronicfatigue/
    mbody.htm

Source: 1
Navigation: 2
Interactivity: 1
Overall: 2

This is a large accumulation of health information on CFS. Some of it is original content from About.com, while some is on other websites to which this one links. Look at the URL (address) to determine if you're reading original content or linked information (About.com will still be in the address if you are on the home site). This site offers a lot of health information, so it's worth checking out. Do be careful about the sources, and prepare to be bombarded with e-commerce appeals.

Ask NOAH About: Chronic Fatigue Syndrome and
  Fibromyalgia
www.noah-health.org/english/illness/neuro/cfs.html#
  Basic%20Descriptions

Source: 1
Navigation: 2
Interactivity: 1
Overall: 1

This site provides a wealth of information, as it pulls together
articles, news, facts, statistics, and more from the Web. There is
one huge disclaimer, however: most of the content is simply
links to other websites. This is a smart strategy because "Asking NOAH" results in a tremendous amount of information on
CFS. Visit this site, and you'll probably find what you're looking for. You must be vigilant about the information on the sites
you end up on. Most seem to be fairly credible, but look at the
URL (address) often to see where you really are.

The CFIDS/M.E. Information Page
www.cfids-me.org

Source: 1
Navigation: 2
Interactivity: 1
Overall: 2

A website by and for people with chronic fatigue and immune
dysfunction syndrome (CFIDS). It's not visually appealing as
it's just a set of links to internal and external Internet resources.
Still, there's a lot of information here (notably other CFS resources, jumbled together in a rather unorganized fashion).
However, it's always helpful to read the advice of others who

share your condition or illness and where they think you should look for more information. Check it out. It's got a lot to offer, just don't expect anything pretty, neat, or right there to educate you about CFS—you'll have to travel a bit.

Cheney Clinic Information Services
www.fnmedcenter.com/ccis

Source: 3
Navigation: 2
Interactivity: 1
Overall: 2

The Glossary and FAQs provide some health education for the site user, but the real feature that makes this site unique is that you can take a Chronic Fatigue Syndrome Probability Test. This test should be used only for educational and screening purposes, not as a sole means of diagnosing chronic fatigue syndrome. Ironically, the site does not have a great deal of basic information on the disorder.

The Chronic Fatigue and Immune Dysfunction
  Syndrome Association of America
www.cfids.org

Source: 3
Navigation: 3
Interactivity: 1
Overall: 3

Even though there are no interactive features (except for a vote), I still give this site a top rating. It's refreshing to find a top-notch site devoted to the condition and its sufferers. There are information about CFS, tips, news, tremendous resources (for many different people who might visit the site), advocacy group listings, and more. If you're suffering from CFS or know someone who is, this is the site to visit!

Chronic Fatigue Syndrome/Myalgic Encephalomyelitis
www.cfs-news.org

Source: 2
Navigation: 2
Interactivity: 1
Overall: 2

This is a great place to visit to get CFS links for news, feature articles, discussion groups, and links to CFS websites around the world. Most of the site is just that—links—but that could be great if you're seeking further resources and information. There appears to be very little original (educational) content on the site, so visit in order to go to outside resources rather than to be educated right there.

MEDLINEplus on Chronic Fatigue Syndrome
www.nlm.nih.gov/medlineplus/
    chronicfatiguesyndrome.html

Source: 3
Navigation: 3
Interactivity: 1
Overall: 2

From the National Institutes of Health, this site is a highly credible, comprehensive resource for those seeking information on CFS. It covers the disease, its management, treatment, directories, and other topics. Linking visitors out to other appropriate NIH resources, as well as those of the CDC, it maintains its high credibility. It is streamlined and simple and provides the basics and beyond.

National Center for Infectious Diseases on Chronic Fatigue Syndrome
www.cdc.gov/ncidod/diseases/cfs

Source: 3
Navigation: 3
Interactivity: 1
Overall: 2

The National Center for Infectious Diseases of the Centers for Disease Control has created this website devoted to CFS. Extremely credible and easy to navigate (it's quite small), this site is a good place to visit when seeking top-line information, treatment options, support groups, research, and publications on the condition. It's thorough, credible, and user-friendly.

National Institute of Allergy and Infectious Diseases on Chronic Fatigue Syndrome
www.niaid.nih.gov/publications/cfs.htm

Source: 3
Navigation: 2
Interactivity: 1
Overall: 2

This should be your first stop when looking for information on CFS. There's solid science behind the data, and the information is presented in an easy-to-read format. This site has something for everyone, so just find what suits you and read carefully. There aren't a great number of links, but the site does hook you into the latest research and news. Get the ABCs here before you move out to other Net resources.

New Jersey Chronic Fatigue Syndrome
    & Fibromyalgia Center
www.umdnj.edu/cfsweb/CFS/cfshome.html

Source: 2
Navigation: 2
Interactivity: 1
Overall: 1

There's not much on this site—but you'll find fairly credible information. The FAQs could go a long way for an inquiring visitor.

Chronic Obstructive Pulmonary Disease
See **Respiratory Diseases/Emphysema/Chronic Obstructive Pulmonary Disease**

Cirrhosis
See **Liver/Cirrhosis.**

Dermatology/Skin Disorders

AcneNet
www.skincarephysicians.com/acnenet

Source: 3
Navigation: 3

Interactivity: 1
Overall: 2

This site is a collaborative effort by Roche Laboratories and the American Academy of Dermatology. However, even though the information on the site is sponsored by an unrestricted educational grant from Roche Laboratories, no flagrant pushing of medications created by this company is apparent. The site is an excellent resource for patients trying to obtain information on the causes, implications, and treatments of acne. A glossary of terms is very helpful, as are the "Basic facts about acne," "Why and how it happens," treatment recommendations, and information about the social impact of acne.

AgingSkinNet
www.skincarephysicians.com/agingskinnet

Source: 3
Navigation: 2
Interactivity: 1
Overall: 3

This is an educational website created by the American Academy of Dermatology and funded by an unrestricted grant from Ortho Dermatological. The focus is on the effects of aging, smoking, sun, and other environmental factors on the skin, and what treatments are available to reverse the signs of aging. This is an excellent site for an older population, as it covers topics such as spider veins, skin cancers, hair loss, and aging skin as well as treatments for each of these conditions. It's easy to navigate (in spite of the absence of a search function), clearly written, and highly credible, coming from the AAD. There is no pushing of products by the supporting pharmaceutical company either. I like it—and so would my mom.

American Academy of Dermatology
www.aad.org/patient_intro.html

Source: 3
Navigation: 3
Interactivity: 1
Overall: 3

A very clear and well organized site from the American Academy of Dermatology that offers resources and tools for those seeking information and access to care. It would benefit from at least *some* free and useful patient education on skin care and disorders; however, the visitor is diverted to subsites (which are actually excellent, by the way, and make my top 10). An excellent section of the website, devoted to children, is called "Kids' Connection"; it teaches kids about healthy skin care at an early age.

DermatologyChannel
www.dermatologychannel.net

Source: 3
Navigation: 3
Interactivity: 3
Overall: 3

This site is developed and staffed by physicians, and offers a comprehensive source for those seeking information on skin care issues. It covers the major dermatology conditions, with facts, treatments, FAQs, and news about each. The community features are also extensive, including how to find a doctor, an "ask a doctor" option, a medical store, a bookstore, and live chats. DermatologyChannel is one of currently fifteen "channels" created by Healthcommunities.com, which features other sites ranging from AlternativeMedicineChannel to

WomensHealthChannel. It's full of information and tools and has my endorsement.

EarthDerm.com
www.earthderm.com
Or go directly to: www.skin-disease.com

Source: 1
Navigation: 1
Interactivity: 1
Overall: 1

This is a good site from which to gather information and treatment recommendations (strongly emphasized) for many skin conditions. It's not pretty to look at, and it's somewhat confusing with many collateral sites, but it's still a solid place to learn the basics on various conditions and how to treat them. Add it to your list of places to search, but don't make it your only stop.

EczemaNet
www.skincarephysicians.com/eczemanet/index.htm

Source: 3
Navigation: 1
Interactivity: 1
Overall: 2

This is an educational site created by the American Academy of Dermatology through an unrestricted educational grant from Fujisawa Healthcare. For those seeking information on eczema and treatment options, this is a great place to visit. Like the other AAD subsites, this is easy to understand and friendly to surf, providing the basics (and beyond) in a cheerful yet credible, user-friendly manner. I particularly like the section "Healthy Skin Tips."

> National Institute of Arthritis and Musculoskeletal and Skin Diseases
> www.nih.gov/niams/healthinfo
>
> *Source: 3*
> *Navigation: 1*
> *Interactivity: 1*
> *Overall: 1*

I wanted to add this site to this list because virtually nothing is more credible than the National Institutes of Health. This site is good for searching because it offers a strong database of information and search options—but you have to know what you're looking for. There could and should be more information on this site. Nonetheless, use it as a resource to link to more information and sources. You can contact NIAMS about specifics or find out about coalitions near you.

> NZ DermNet
> www.dermnet.org.nz
>
> *Source: 3*
> *Navigation: 3*
> *Interactivity: 1*
> *Overall: 3*

The website of the New Zealand Dermatological Society aims to provide authoritative information about the skin for health professionals and patients with skin diseases. The best place to check out is the section for patients. The information about skin diseases is written for interested patients rather than experts and is easy to follow. The clean, clear home page and layout almost feel like clean, clear skin.

PsoriasisNet
www.skincarephysicians.com/psoriasisnet/index.htm

Source: 3
Navigation: 1
Interactivity: 1
Overall: 2

This is an educational site created by the American Academy of Dermatology through an unrestricted educational grant from Fujisawa Healthcare. For those seeking information on psoriasis and its treatment options, this is an excellent site to check out. It's easy to navigate, informative, and highly credible—what else could one ask for?

Diabetes

American Diabetes Association
www.diabetes.org

Source: 3
Navigation: 2
Interactivity: 2
Overall: 3

The American Diabetes Association is a world-renowned organization leading the charge in education about the disease and advocacy for diabetics. The site, however, can be a little chaotic with all of the organizational announcements in the right-hand margin that constantly distract your eye. The information is nicely listed in the left-hand margin, and you can find out about issues from exercise to special diabetic recipes. Despite being "busy," the site is easy to navigate. It also offers the information in Spanish. One neat trick is that it allows you to customize the site to your specifications.

Canadian Diabetes Association
www.diabetes.ca

Source: 3
Navigation: 3
Interactivity: 1
Overall: 2

The statistics offered by this site, of course, are from Canada, but the information about diabetes is as relevant as anything else you will find on the Internet. The Canadian Diabetes Association, a counterpart to the American Diabetes Association, provides excellent, well-presented diabetes information. The left-hand margin of the home page is full of links to specific information—everything from understanding what insulin is to knowing what food choices are best for diabetics. The links to other Net resources are extensive. This is an excellent source for all levels of those searching for diabetes info.

Centers for Disease Control and Prevention: Diabetes
    Public Health Resource
www.cdc.gov/diabetes

Source: 3
Navigation: 3
Interactivity: 1
Overall: 2

The CDC, in its typically thorough fashion, has delivered a resource page full of everything you might want to know about diabetes. And if it doesn't have what you're looking for, you're sure to find it through its assortment of links. In a way that's unique to the CDC, you're given statistics and a broad perspective on diabetes and its complications. Check out the FAQs, which take you through the basics; when you're done with those, read the latest headlines. These resource pages show once again why the CDC is one of the best providers of disease information on the Net.

Children with Diabetes
www.childrenwithdiabetes.com

Source: 2
Navigation: 3
Interactivity: 2
Overall: 2

This site addresses exactly the demographic in its title, children with diabetes. Parents will find tons of information ranging from the basics of diabetes to the social and family issues that arise when a child is diagnosed. I was surprised to see how well referenced the information was, rather than being just a collection of personal anecdotes. A special feature of the site is weekly chats and particularly the teen chat, which allows young people with diabetes to share their experiences. This is a must-visit site for any parent or child with diabetes.

diabetesonestop.com
www.diabetesonestop.com

Source: 2
Navigation: 2
Interactivity: 1
Overall: 1

This site bills itself as one-stop shopping, which might be a little overstated but is nonetheless well intentioned. You can certainly see the difference between this site and some of the stronger governmental sites. One of the major reasons I've included it is because of its extensive list of links to outside organizations and resources. These links take you all over the world to provide you with the latest in diabetes information. Don't come to this site for the basics, but the site will be quite helpful in navigating the world of diabetes on the Net.

HealthAtoZ.com on Diabetes
www.healthatoz.com/atoz/Diabetes2/diabetesindex2.asp

Source: 2
Navigation: 3
Interactivity: 2
Overall: 2

There's a lot of diabetes information on the Internet, but HealthAtoZ.com compacts it and gives you the most important. The site has nicely divided diabetes into its two major subtypes, I and II, and takes you through what you need to know in a well-organized, easy-to-navigate way. A special feature of the site is the diary that helps you keep track of your blood sugar levels, weight, exercise, and mealtimes. The site also gives you the latest diabetes news headlines, right next to the basics. Its message board is a fun way to hear from others battling the same disease. This is a friendly, low-key website that will quench your thirst for diabetes information.

Joslin Diabetes Center
www.joslin.harvard.edu

Source: 2
Navigation: 3
Interactivity: 2
Overall: 2

This website, which is affiliated with the Harvard Medical School, is just what you would expect from such a prestigious institution. It is full of excellent information that is written in a way for all to understand. Whether you're a beginner or a health professional, this site will answer your needs. It provides information as basic as what diabetes is and how it's commonly treated to news of the latest research. It also offers a discussion board to communicate with other diabetics. Whether you are a newly diagnosed patient or a researcher, you can't miss with this site.

Juvenile Diabetes Foundation International
www.jdrf.org

Source: 3
Navigation: 2
Interactivity: 2
Overall: 2

When you log on to the JDF's home page, you immediately feel the power of the organization. The website is a mix of advocacy, breaking research news, and basic information on type I diabetes. There is so much information on the home page that you almost don't need to go anywhere else. A special feature of the site is its "Clinical trials" link, which gives you not only the latest information on clinical trials throughout the world but a chance to join one if there is one near you. For parents with children diagnosed with type I diabetes, not stopping at this website would be a big mistake.

National Kidney Foundation
www.kidney.org

Source: 2
Navigation: 1

Interactivity: 1
Overall: 1

The site of the National Kidney Foundation is a solid provider of basic information about diabetes and some of its complications. It will not blow you away with fancy graphics or a long list of links. Diabetes is only one of several kidney diseases it covers, and it does so succinctly and without much hoopla. You will likely visit a more specialized diabetes site after surfing these pages, but you will undoubtedly be seduced by its information on other kidney disorders. Stop by for sure, but don't make it your last stop.

National Institute of Diabetes & Digestive & Kidney
   Diseases
www.niddk.nih.gov

Source: 3
Navigation: 3
Interactivity: 1
Overall: 3

This is one of the best websites that addresses diabetes and all of its related complications. As is typical with most government sites, it doesn't bother you with distracting advertising or logos. Instead, it's neatly organized, easy to read, fun to navigate, and so full of information that after surfing the site you might not want to go anywhere else because of information overload. The information is updated frequently and, as far as credibility is concerned, how about having the most distinguished researchers in the world providing information? This is how a health website should be constructed!

Emphysema
See **Respiratory Diseases/Emphysema/Chronic Obstructive Pulmonary Disease.**

Endocrinology
(Thyroid, parathyroid, adrenal, and pancreas disorders; also see **Diabetes.**)

American Association of Clinical Endocrinologists
www.aace.com

Source: 3
Navigation: 1
Interactivity: 1
Overall: 1

This site is definitely not for the Internet beginner. While there is good information available, heavy navigation is required to uncover it. Part of the site is restricted to members, who must be physicians. However, the information available to the public is extremely comprehensive and credible, if a little on the advanced side. I'm not fond of the advertising on the home page, but fortunately it appears at the bottom, where it's least intrusive. You can find an endocrinologist near you or work to manage your diabetes online with a support team. Don't come here first for the basics, but if you're up to the challenge, you won't be disappointed.

CliniWeb International on Endocrine Diseases
www.ohsu.edu/cliniweb/C19/C19.html

Source: 1
Navigation: 2

Interactivity: N/A
Overall: 1

This site is really just a long list of information links. The organization isn't the greatest, and the site could be constructed to
be more user-friendly. That said, there is an enormous amount
of information available about a variety of topics. The content
on this site is drawn from experts and institutions from around
the world. If you are willing to sort through a lot of links, this
site could take your Net fancy. Interactive tools would make
this site a lot more useful, but because the content is so broad
and the information is so good, I'm not deterred from recom-
mending it.

Columbia University College of Physicians and Surgeons
http://cpmcnet.columbia.edu/texts/guide/toc/toc21.html

Source: 2
Navigation: 3
Interactivity: 1
Overall: 1

This is part of Columbia University College's home medical
guide written specifically with consumers in mind. The site
covers a wide range of endocrine disorders and delivers the
information in an easy-to-read format. You won't be distracted by advertisements. This is a chapter of the guide,
rather than a complete website dedicated to endocrine disorders. Nonetheless, the info it contains is not so in-depth as to
scare away the beginner nor so simple as to turn away those
already knowledgeable about the disorder. There's a better
than good chance that you'll find information on the disease
you're researching.

EndocrineWeb.com
www.endocrineweb.com

Source: 3
Navigation: 3
Interactivity: 3
Overall: 3

Not only does this site offer excellent information on a wide range of endocrine disorders, it also has links to an exemplary group of links to other endocrine resources. The interactive tools on this site set it apart from the rest. You can read and post information on the message board or chat online with physicians or others with a similar medical experience. There's also an online support group you can join to better understand issues related to your disease. This site offers you one of the best-rounded experiences in researching endocrinology information.

The Endocrine Society
www.endo-society.org

Source: 3
Navigation: 3
Interactivity: 1
Overall: 2

This is the first and possibly only stop you will need in your quest for information on endocrine disorders. It's the website of one of the country's most respected endocrine organizations. The fact sheets located in the patient information section are not only comprehensive but easy to read. You can find information on the rarest of diseases to the most common, such as diabetes. There are great links to external resources. You can also read the latest endocrinology headlines. If more websites were designed like this, your searches and my job writing this book would be much easier.

Karolinska Institute Endocrine Links
www.mic.ki.se/Diseases/c19.html

Source: 2
Navigation: 3
Interactivity: 3
Overall: 3

This site is simply a place to find links to other sites dealing with endocrinology. This Swedish institute has made its website available in English. The list of links is long and one of the most comprehensive that I've seen on the Net. If you're stuck trying to find a place to visit, try this site and see all of the wonderful resources you can access. This is not a place to get basic information on a particular endocrine disease, nor does it pretend to be, but it will help you find answers to any specific questions you may have.

National Institute of Diabetes & Digestive & Kidney
    Diseases on Endocrine and Metabolic Disorders
www.niddk.nih.gov/health/endo/endo.htm

Source: 3
Navigation: 3
Interactivity: 1
Overall: 3

This site is a hands-down winner. It's backed by the best in science, and it's organized as every site should be. It's also easy on the eyes and fingers. The FAQs tend to be general, but they're also linked to more specific sites, and the site as a whole links to outside resources that can also provide valuable information.

If you have limited time and can hit only a few sites, this should definitely be one of them. It doesn't deal with all of the endocrine disorders, but it certainly covers the main ones.

UpToDate in Endocrinology and Diabetes
www.uptodate.com/html/prendo.htm

Source: 2
Navigation: 3
Interactivity: 1
Overall: 2

If you want to know the tone and intentions of this site, read the bottom of the home page. This may not do a lot to fill its coffers, but it does a world of good for consumers. First, you're not bombarded with bothersome ads, and second, you know that the site concentrates on delivering quality information. This is an excellent source of endocrinology information that will immediately increase your understanding of the disorder that most concerns you. You will have access to an extensive drug database and a summary of the latest advances. You'll find good, reliable information in abundance here.

Epilepsy

American Academy of Neurology
www.aan.com

Source: 3
Navigation: 2
Interactivity: 1
Overall: 2

The American Academy of Neurology is one of the most respected neurological organizations in the country. It deals with a range of conditions, including epilepsy. Its site has excellent patient brochures and information about this condition. It also lists several links to outside resources and sites. There is little interactivity, but the information is of first-rate quality that you can trust.

British Epilepsy Association
www.epilepsy.org.uk

Source: 2
Navigation: 3
Interactivity: 3
Overall: 3

This is a complete site on epilepsy. Here you can find excellent information that is comprehensive and easy to read. The interactive tools are equally impressive, allowing you to participate in chats or visit the kids' section. When you've gotten your fill of information, try some of the links that will send you to sites around the globe.

Comprehensive Epilepsy Center of New York Hospital
http://neuro.med.cornell.edu/NYH-CMC/
    n-epilepsy.html

Source: 2
Navigation: 3
Interactivity: 1
Overall: 2

If you want no-frills, reliable information on epilepsy, this is your place. There aren't any advertisements or solicitations. These serious academic physicians are giving you the facts without excess. You'll appreciate not only the completeness of the information, but how it's written for you to understand without having to keep a medical dictionary nearby. There are no truly interactive tools, but the intention of this site is to provide information, which it does quickly and well.

Epilepsy.com
www.epilepsy.com

Source: 2
Navigation: 3
Interactivity: 3
Overall: 3

This site is so full of epilepsy information you could drown in it. The writing is elegant and easy to read and the layout so well organized you could navigate it in your sleep. Take advantage of the live chats and the message boards to discuss epilepsy with others who have suffered from or been involved with it. Also, read some of the inspiring stories of others who have battled the disease and continue to win.

Epilepsy Foundation
www.efa.org

Source: 3
Navigation: 3
Interactivity: 3
Overall: 3

This is undoubtedly one of the best epilepsy sites on the Net. It's full of important information and written in a way that can be understood by everyone. The site is organized into several sections, including ones for adults, women, parents, seniors, and teens. You'll be amazed by the quality of the content and the detail in which it describes the condition and its treatments. The e-community and its interactive chats and forums are excellent places to exchange information and get feedback on epilepsy issues.

KidsHealth
www.kidshealth.org/parent/medical/brain/epilepsy.html

Source: 3
Navigation: 2
Interactivity: 2
Overall: 2

This site is dedicated to kids' health, and the pages on epilepsy cover the issue from every angle. You can read excellent articles that have been marked for parents, teens, and kids. If you want to read more about epilepsy because the site hasn't given you enough info, just click on to one of the many links to other Net resources.

MEDLINEplus on Epilepsy
www.nlm.nih.gov/medlineplus/epilepsy.html

Source: 3
Navigation: 3
Interactivity: 1
Overall: 2

This is a site that would be a great first stop in your search for epilepsy information. The information is simply presented and easy to understand, and the site covers a broad spectrum of epilepsy-related information. The links to other websites connect you to other valuable information sources. This is a great source of information and an entry point to the rest of the epilepsy information on the Web.

National Institute of Neurological Disorders and Stroke on Epilepsy
www.ninds.nih.gov/health_and_medical/disorders/
epilepsy.htm

Source: 3
Navigation: 3
Interactivity: 1
Overall: 2

This is the government's site on neurological disorders and prominently includes epilepsy and related issues. The information is plentiful and easy to understand. The site is uncluttered, making navigation a cinch. Reading through these pages will increase your knowledge of epilepsy exponentially.

NeurologyChannel
www.neurologychannel.com

Source: 3
Navigation: 3
Interactivity: 3
Overall: 3

If you want to learn about epilepsy, you might not need to look any further than this site. The information is comprehensive, well written, and easy to understand. The site is your complete guide to epilepsy information that includes live chats, an "Ask the Doctor" link, and a "Find the Doctor" tool. If you have time to research only a few sites, this should be one of them.

Fibromyalgia

American Fibromyalgia Syndrome Association, Inc.
www.afsafund.org

Source: 2
Navigation: 2
Interactivity: 1
Overall: 1

This site is best used if you're looking for the latest research or updates regarding fibromyalgia. You won't necessarily get the ABCs of fibromyalgia but rather different articles and headlines on the disease. There is also quite an extensive list of resources that could assist in your search for information or help you battle the disease. This site is for someone looking for more than just the basics.

Arthritis Foundation on Fibromyalgia
www.arthritis.org/conditions/drugguide/fibromyalgia_
    about.asp

Source: 3
Navigation: 3
Interactivity: 2
Overall: 2

This site contains straightforward information on the basics of fibromyalgia. It's written with the consumer in mind. The site is also simple in design, making it easy to navigate. You are given a couple of resources at the bottom of the page that can also be helpful. This is good place to start learning the basics.

Chronic Fatigue Syndrome & Fibromyalgia Information
  Exchange Forum
www.co-cure.org

Source: 1
Navigation: 2
Interactivity: 1
Overall: 2

This organization lists as one of its major missions the exchange of fibromyalgia information among patients, doctors, political organizations, and other institutions. The site is designed to draw on several sources and direct you to many others. You will find information, but you'll have to work a little. Be patient; you will be rewarded for your diligence.

familydoctor.org on Fibromyalgia
www.familydoctor.org/handouts/070.html

Source: 3
Navigation: 2
Interactivity: 1
Overall: 2

This site, which belongs to the American Academy of Family Physicians, is designed to provide credible information that's relevant and easy to read. The search engine is excellent and will retrieve a vast amount of information related to fibromyalgia and its diagnosis and treatment. A lot of your questions will be answered on the site's many informative pages.

Fibromyalgia Patient Support Center
www.fmpsc.org

Source: 1
Navigation: 3

Interactivity: 3
Overall: 2

This site is excellent for patient-to-patient communication. It contains a wide range of information and services and connects you to fibromyalgia sources around the World Wide Web. The information isn't always written by experts, so that must be taken into account when evaluating the information's credibility. The strength of this website is its seemingly endless supply of support information and the extensive list of resources. If you're a patient, this is one place you should stop to learn what help there may be out there for you.

MayoClinic.com on Fibromyalgia
www.mayoclinic.com/home?id=5.1.1.6.5

Source: 3
Navigation: 3
Interactivity: 2
Overall: 3

This is one of the best fibromyalgia sources on the Net. The information is extremely credible and presented in a manner for all to understand. You can navigate the site with the smallest amount of effort, and there's so much information here that you can't help but leave the site better informed. The additional resources listed at the bottom of the page would be great to continue your search for information.

Missouri Arthritis Rehabilitation Research and Training
    Center on Fibromyalgia
www.hsc.missouri.edu/~fibro

Source: 3
Navigation: 3

Interactivity: 1
Overall: 3

This site is pleasantly designed and easy to navigate. The information is simple and written for all to understand. You will get quite a lesson on fibromyalgia by surfing through the site's pages. The information is credible, and the list of fibromyalgia links is most impressive; these other resources can satisfy whatever questions you still have after navigating this site. This is a must-stop site for fibromyalgia information.

National Fibromyalgia Awareness Campaign
www.fmaware.com

Source: 2
Navigation: 3
Interactivity: 1
Overall: 2

Basic information is ready for you on this site. You'll get a quick lesson in fibromyalgia that will inform and guide you with little effort. You'll also be able to access a list of links that can lead you to other Net sources on the disease. The organization's goal is to raise awareness, and this site certainly provides the facts to do so.

National Institute of Arthritis and Musculoskeletal and
    Skin Diseases
www.nih.gov/niams/healthinfo/fibrofs.htm

Source: 3
Navigation: 3
Interactivity: 1
Overall: 1

This is a U.S. government site that provides information on fibromyalgia. The content is simple and not as in-depth as other sites, but it covers the basics quickly. There aren't any links to other sites, but a very useful list of organizational resources and their numbers is provided. You won't learn all you need to know on fibromyalgia, but you'll get a good idea of what the disease is all about.

MEDLINEplus on Fibromyalgia
www.nlm.nih.gov/medlineplus/fibromyalgia.html

Source: 3
Navigation: 3
Interactivity: 1
Overall: 2

This site is like an encyclopedia that allows you to search for and find information on fibromyalgia. This information is drawn from a variety of sources and is easy to read. The site is simple to navigate and uncluttered by advertisements or advocacy solicitations. If you're interested in research articles, this site allows you to retrieve a great number of them. If you speak Spanish, this site will suit your fancy also. This is an excellent source for fibromyalgia information.

Fitness
See **Sports Medicine/Fitness.**

Gynecology
See **Obstetrics and Gynecology.**

Hair Loss

American Academy of Dermatology on Hair Loss
www.aad.org/pamphlets/hairloss.html

Source: 3
Navigation: 3
Interactivity: 1
Overall: 1

Here you'll find thoughtful information presented simply. It belongs to the most prestigious academy of experts who deal with hair loss; thus you would expect more than what it delivers. There is a search engine that can help you find a dermatologist nearest you, but other than that, there are not many extras. You can stop here to read about hair loss, but you will need to visit other sites before your hunt is over.

American Hair Loss Council
www.ahlc.org

Source: 2
Navigation: 3
Interactivity: 1
Overall: 2

This site focuses on reversing hair loss and preventing more of your valued hairs from falling out. It does, however, offer some basic information on the different types and causes of hair loss. There is a search engine that helps you look for a specialist in your area. These specialists are members of the Hair Loss Council and have been certified as hair loss specialists. This qualification, however, should not be the only criterion you use when choosing a doctor to address your hair loss. You won't get the most information here, but enough to get an understanding of what's going on and how you can treat it.

Best Doctors on Hair Loss
www.bestdoctors.com/en/askadoctor/c/cohen/bhcohen_
   052200.htm

Source: 2
Navigation: 2
Interactivity: 1
Overall: 1

This site won't wow you, but it will provide you with solid information about hair loss and its treatment. Most of the answers are provided by a leading expert, who presents the information in a question-and-answer format. This site covers the basics without a lot of preliminaries, giving you the information you need in readable language and efficiently. This shouldn't be your only stop while searching for information, but it should be included with the others.

Follicle.com
www.follicle.com

Source: 1
Navigation: 3
Interactivity: 1
Overall: 1

I like this site a lot. However, it doesn't provide enough information about the contributors and their credentials. Nonetheless, the information is presented in a logical, well-organized manner. Of particular interest is the explanation of hair growth and structure and the picture that accompanies it. You'll leave this site with a very good understanding of how our hair grows and the factors that contribute to its loss.

Healthology on Hair Loss
www.healthology.com/focus_index.asp?f=hairloss

Source: 2
Navigation: 3
Interactivity: 2
Overall: 2

This is an excellent site for people trying to understand the basics of why age seems to zap away the hairs from our head. The contributors are mainly physicians and credentialed health professionals. There are several interesting features about this site, including webcasts from some of the most prominent hair loss specialists in the world. There are also well-written, easy-to-understand articles that cover a wide range of issues related to hair loss. This is a must-visit site for anyone looking for answers about the balding process.

HeliosHealth.com on Male Pattern Baldness
www.helioshealth.com/mpb

Source: 3
Navigation: 3
Interactivity: 2
Overall: 3

You can't help but like this site as soon as you log on. It's well organized, features the questions that you want to ask, and provides the answers to those questions. The information is presented logically and without much in the way of doctor-speak so that you can understand what's happening. The site explains what causes hair loss, then takes you through some of the options for preventing further loss or replacing what has already disappeared. While surfing the site, check the message board and see what others have to say about their hair loss and treatment.

Keratin.com
www.keratin.com

Source: 3
Navigation: 3
Interactivity: 3
Overall: 3

If you're going to search for hair loss information on the Net, this is definitely the place to start. The home page is the best I've seen for those looking for answers about why their hair is falling out and what can be done to stop the process or replace the hair. It has everything you could possibly want. It's by far the best-rounded hair loss site you'll find. You can read and post messages on the board; participate in and read the results of anonymous surveys; learn about specific conditions that cause hair loss; and read about the treatment options. If you don't stop here for hair loss information, you could be making a big mistake.

MoreHair.com
www.morehair.com

Source: 1
Navigation: 3
Interactivity: 3
Overall: 2

This site is full of important hair loss information. You can read about the different types of hair loss and the various treatments available to prevent more from falling out. The writing is simple but effective. You can also be part of an online forum that discusses different subjects concerning hair loss. This shouldn't be the first place to visit on your Net tour but it wouldn't hurt to stop by, especially if you want to participate in an online conversation on the topic.

National Alopecia Areata Foundation
www.alopeciaareata.com

Source: 3
Navigation: 3
Interactivity: 2
Overall: 2

This site deals specifically with alopecia areata, an autoimmune skin disorder that causes hair loss from the scalp and the rest of the body. It is an excellent site that provides important information about what the disease is and what treatments are available. You can also hear from others who suffer from the same illness by visiting the message board. If alopecia areata is your diagnosis, this is the place to find out more.

Regrowth.com
www.regrowth.com

Source: 1
Navigation: 3
Interactivity: 3
Overall: 2

I've included this site for three reasons. One: You can get the latest headlines on hair loss. Two: The interactive options are excellent, allowing you to chat with others and participate in discussion forums. Three: Its excellent list of links is neatly organized. The editorial guidelines and review process aren't explained well, so the fact sheets must be used cautiously. However, the other offerings of the site are enough for a stopover.

Headache

The Headache and Migraine Information Site
www.headache.com.au

Source: 3
Navigation: 2
Interactivity: 2
Overall: 2

Right off, this site isn't very friendly, but it's helpful. It's also designed with the Australian headache sufferer in mind, though it's obviously useful on the other side of the Pacific as well. The site's strongest point is its detailed breakdown of bodily regions (particularly those above the neck) that cause headaches. Grab a comfy chair, because the site is rather slow.

Headache Cybertext
www.upstate.edu/neurology/haas

Source: 3
Navigation: 2
Interactivity: 1
Overall: 2

This is an information-rich site. However, its intended audience is physicians and medical students. If you're willing to give it time and read a sentence over two or three times, it can be of help in pinpointing exactly what type of headache you're experiencing and how it can be treated.

HealingWell.com: Migraine-Headache Resource Center
www.healingwell.com/migraines

Source: 2
Navigation: 2
Interactivity: 2
Overall: 2

Don't let the title fool you—this website is about more than just migraines. It is information-packed and pulls its content from various sources. A professional yet friendly site, it covers a huge range of diagnosis and treatments—just try not to feel overwhelmed.

HealthCentral.com on Headaches & Migraines
www.healthcentral.com/Centers/OneCenter.cfm?Center=
    Migraines

Source: 2
Navigation: 2
Interactivity: 2
Overall: 2

This site has a lot of information about headaches. There are books, articles, and other Internet resources to further explore on this site. And the active Dr. Dean Edell can be counted on to provide a lively discussion. The navigation of the site could be improved. One can get a little frustrated with the multiple clicks and the small font. You won't find the site aesthetically pleasing and that extra click might annoy you, but there's excellent information here to compensate for your effort.

MEDLINEplus on Headache and Migraine
www.nlm.nih.gov/medlineplus/headacheandmigraine.html

Source: 3
Navigation: 3

Interactivity: 1
Overall: 3

This is a good example of a one-stop site. It pulls its content
from various sources, a useful technique when the sufferers include children and seniors, for whom there is not a great deal of
headache information. Like other MEDLINEplus pages, this
one also includes some information for Spanish speakers.

National Headache Foundation
www.headaches.org

Source: 2
Navigation: 2
Interactivity: 1
Overall: 2

Admittedly, this website takes some maneuvering around to
find the information you want. But once you're in the education section, doors begin to open in relation to your headache questions. It's a nonprofit organization that you can also
join. It's filled with interesting facts and is dedicated, as its
name implies, to helping people who must cope with recur-
ring headaches.

National Institute of Neurological Disorders and Stroke
    on Headaches
www.ninds.nih.gov/health_and_medical/pubs/headache_
    htr.htm

Source: 3
Navigation: 3
Interactivity: 1
Overall: 2

Many of the most common questions regarding headaches are answered with the click of a mouse, even without scrolling. The sample scenarios highlight what some headache sufferers go through. This helps visitors to the site connect with others who've experienced similar pain. A glossary gives words and definitions to help sufferers name their conditions rather than merely describe the problem. The site won't floor you with its look, but you should find it helpful.

Neurology Channel
www.neurologychannel.com/headache

Source: 3
Navigation: 3
Interactivity: 3
Overall: 3

One of the best resources on the Internet for headaches is the Neurology Channel. The information is straightforward and highly useful. In addition to answering questions about the pain's source(s), it takes you from identifying the symptoms to finding the best and proper treatment. The site provides an opportunity to have fun while seeking answers.

PageWise
http://nmnm.essortment.com/headacherelief_nus.htm

Source: 1
Navigation: 3
Interactivity: 1
Overall: 1

This is a perfect site for the person who has a headache and is about to reach for the medicine cabinet. There are many web-sites on headaches that are more detailed, some less, and some have about the same amount of information as this one. The language on this site, however, is designed for the average person who has a headache from time to time and wants to know why, how they happen, and what can be done. The site doesn't frighten you with its contents, but it does warn that you might need to seek out a physician.

Heart Disease

American Heart Association National Center
www.americanheart.org

Source: 3
Navigation: 3
Interactivity: 1
Overall: 3

If you are looking for heart information from A to Z, this is the site for you. It contains comprehensive, easy-to-read information on a variety of heart diseases and their treatment and, most important, tips on prevention.

Ask NOAH About: Heart Disease and Stroke
www.noah-health.org/english/illness/heart_disease/
    heartdisease.html

Source: 3
Navigation: 2

Interactivity: 2
Overall: 2

Those who enjoy one-stop shopping will love this site! It contains links to an amazing number of credible sites, organized by topic and covering basic to advanced information on heart disease, its care and treatment, support groups, statistics, and even the *U.S. News & World Report* hospital ratings for hospitals that specialize in cardiovascular disease.

Children's Health Information Network on Congenital
    Heart Disease
www.tchin.org

Source: 2
Navigation: 3
Interactivity: 2
Overall: 2

This is a great resource not only for information on congenital heart disease, but also for moral support. An expert advisory panel lends credibility to the site, which also contains an inspirational "Memorial Garden" containing the life stories of children who have died of congenital and acquired heart disease.

The Franklin Institute Online
www.sln.fi.edu/biosci/preview/heartpreview.html

Source: 2
Navigation: 3
Interactivity: 3
Overall: 2

If you want to take an online tour of the heart, this fascinating site allows you to explore at your own pace. It contains basic information about the heart's anatomy, heart health, and the prevention of heart disease. It's like visiting a museum exhibit (complete with sound effects!) without leaving the comfort of your home.

Heart Information Network
www.heartinfo.org

Source: 2
Navigation: 2
Interactivity: 2
Overall: 2

This site is a good place to start your research on heart disease. It has a great listing of recent news articles and provides a wide range of information and resources for heart patients, including patients' stories organized by the patients' risk factors. Some people may find the library of questions and answers very helpful.

Lifeclinic.com
www.lifeclinic.com

Source: 2
Navigation: 3
Interactivity: 2
Overall: 2

This is a well-organized site containing information on blood pressure, cholesterol, diabetes, and stroke. The site has a strong advisory board, and the information appears to be accurate. But do keep in mind that this is a commercial site; that is, it contains good information but includes a sprinkling of marketing.

MayoClinic.com on Heart Disease
www.mayohealth.org/home?id=3.1.9

Source: 3
Navigation: 3
Interactivity: 2
Overall: 2

This site contains a wealth of information and interactive tools covering the gamut of heart disease. The news section is updated regularly to keep you current on trends and advances in cardiovascular disease.

Medem
www.medem.com

Source: 3
Navigation: 3
Interactivity: 1
Overall: 3

This is a well-organized site with information geared toward patients and professionals, allowing you to begin with the basics and move on to more advanced technical information if you like. This site is reviewed by board-certified physicians and generally contains only peer-reviewed information, so it can be considered an authoritative source.

National Heart, Lung, and Blood Institute:
    Cardiovascular Information
www.nhlbi.nih.gov/health/public/heart

Source: 3
Navigation: 3
Interactivity: 2
Overall: 3

This is a valuable resource for anyone interested in information about high blood pressure, cholesterol, and obesity and their effects on the heart. It also contains useful heart-healthy recipes and a variety of interactive tools. For African-American researchers, this site has booklets geared specifically toward the particular issues facing African Americans with cardiovascular disease and healthy home-style soul food recipes.

PediHeart
www.pediheart.org

Source: 2
Navigation: 2
Interactivity: 1
Overall: 2

This site is an excellent resource for parents of children with congenital heart disease. The information is well organized and easy to read with graphics that illuminate some of the more complex details. It also has a section for kids with heart disease, containing kid-friendly information and an opportunity to network with other kids for support.

Hepatitis C
(Also see **Liver.**)

American Liver Foundation
www.liverfoundation.org

Source: 3
Navigation: 3
Interactivity: 1
Overall: 3

This site is run by a voluntary, not-for-profit health agency dedicated to research, education, and support related to liver diseases. It contains detailed information not only about hepatitis C but about a variety of other liver diseases. In addition, the site contains advocacy information, white papers, news stories, journal articles, information about alternative medicine treatments, and stories by patients with liver diseases. This is a very elegant and thorough site.

Centers for Disease Control and Prevention on Viral
    Hepatitis C
www.cdc.gov/ncidod/diseases/hepatitis/c

Source: 3
Navigation: 2
Interactivity: 1
Overall: 3

This site contains extensive information about the diagnosis of, testing for, transmission of, and treatment of hepatitis C. It also contains the latest news and surgeon general's recommendations regarding the disease. The site is well organized and easy to navigate but can be slow at times. In addition, some of the information is clearly intended for a professional audience and may be difficult for the average reader to understand.

Hepatitis C Education & Support Network
www.hepcesn.net

Source: 1
Navigation: 2
Interactivity: 1
Overall: 1

This site is sponsored by a grassroots not-for-profit agency. It provides great links to other resources and a detailed listing of support groups. The information content is basically a collection of news and journal articles from a variety of sources, including items e-mailed from visitors to the site, so make sure you carefully review the source of material you are reading.

Hepatitis C Info
www.hepatitiscinfo.com

Source: 2
Navigation: 3
Interactivity: 1
Overall: 2

You'll find this site to be a good source of basic information about hepatitis C. Reliable references add credibility to the information presented.

Hepatitis C Outreach Project
www.hcop.org

Source: 2
Navigation: 2
Interactivity: 1
Overall: 2

This site has a good advisory board, lending credibility to the site. There are easy-to-read informational brochures available for download as well as recent news articles and information regarding liver transplantation.

Hepatitis Foundation International Online
www.hepfi.org

Source: 2
Navigation: 3

Interactivity: 3
Overall: 2

This site contains a variety of information related to hepatitis, including a general overview, treatment options, support groups, tips on coping with the disease, symptoms, causes, and much more. The only caveat is that there is no indication of the original sources of the material presented or mention of any type of editorial board.

The Hepatitis Information Network
www.hepnet.com/hepc.html

Source: 2
Navigation: 3
Interactivity: 2
Overall: 2

This Canadian site features a collection of journal and news articles containing a wide variety of information about all types of hepatitis. Also included is specific information geared to patients and professionals, along with interactive quizzes. The publication dates of the articles are clearly stated so that you know how up-to-date the material is. The content on this site comes from reliable sources, and most of it is peer-reviewed, lending it credibility.

MayoClinic.com on Hepatitis C
www.mayoclinic.com/home?id=5.1.1.8.9

Source: 3
Navigation: 2
Interactivity: 1
Overall: 2

This site is a good place to start for general information about hepatitis C. It is well organized and easy to navigate, but, most important, the information is presented in an easy-to-understand manner. The site was developed and is reviewed regularly by Mayo Clinic physicians and researchers, who add to the credibility of the information.

National Institutes of Health: National Institute of Diabetes and Digestive and Kidney Diseases
www.niddk.nih.gov/health/digest/pubs/chrnhepc/ chrnhepc.htm

Source: 3
Navigation: 3
Interactivity: 2
Overall: 3

This authoritative site, sponsored by the National Institutes of Health, contains good illustrations, primarily educational materials on hepatitis C, and frequently updated information. It's easy to navigate. The information is also available in Spanish.

WebMD
www.webmd.com

Source: 3
Navigation: 3
Interactivity: 1
Overall: 3

This site is a general medical reference site that contains articles and general and advanced information regarding a variety of common illnesses. It is well organized and easy to navigate. Some articles contain illustrations to demystify some of the obscure medical terms. This site has a very good collection of information on hepatitis C.

High Blood Pressure (Hypertension)

American Heart Association on High Blood Pressure
www.americanheart.org

Source: 3
Navigation: 3
Interactivity: 2
Overall: 3

The American Heart Association is the country's leading organization dedicated to treating, raising money for, and educating people about heart disease. The site is well organized, and the information is easy for all to understand. You can test your knowledge of high blood pressure or read up on your risk factors. You'll leave this site a better-informed and (hopefully) healthier person.

American Society of Hypertension
www.ash-us.org

Source: 3
Navigation: 3
Interactivity: 1
Overall: 2

This organization is dedicated to researching and educating people about hypertension. It is sponsored by the best hypertension doctors in the world and draws on this great resource to create an excellent website. Not only will you find basic information about hypertension and the drugs used to treat it, you will also find excellent links to other sites that provide high-quality blood pressure information. This is one of those sites that can both provide substantial information and serve as a launching pad to other Net resources.

CardiologyChannel
www.cardiologychannel.com/hypertension

Source: 2
Navigation: 3
Interactivity: 3
Overall: 3

This site focuses on heart diseases, of which hypertension is one of the most common. It gives you the A-to-Z information and then some. You can navigate it with ease and take advantage of the interactive tools: participate in a live chat or ask the doctor a question. You can also get the latest in blood pressure news and find out if there's a clinical trial that you can join that might help you control the disease better. This might be the only place you need to visit on the Web for blood pressure information.

Hypertension, Dialysis, and Clinical Nephrology
www.hdcn.com

Source: 3
Navigation: 2
Interactivity: 1
Overall: 2

This site provides information about kidney disease and hypertension. Its home page is somewhat cluttered, but with careful navigation you can access important information about hypertension and specific care instructions for different patient populations, such as diabetics or transplant patients. You can also find important information on the latest antihypertensive treatments. This isn't the easiest site on which to find information, but if you're patient it could pay off big time.

Lifeclinic.com on Blood Pressure
www.lifeclinic.com/focus/blood

Source: 2
Navigation: 3
Interactivity: 2
Overall: 2

This colorful site addresses some of the most common heart-related illnesses, including hypertension. It provides important information on the latest treatments and headlines from around the world. There are a lot of interactive tools that allow you to check your risk assessment by recording your blood pressure online and using a health calculator. This site makes taking care of your blood pressure informative but interesting at the same time—something that is not always easy to pull off.

MayoClinic.com on High Blood Pressure
www.mayoclinic.com/home?id=3.1.10

Source: 3
Navigation: 3
Interactivity: 2
Overall: 2

The Mayo Clinic is one of the most respected medical institutions in the world, and this website lives up to its reputation. Here you'll find excellent information on high blood pressure and what you can do to prevent, treat, and control it. Take a quiz to determine your knowledge about and risk of developing high blood pressure, then check out the links to other resources that can also provide help in understanding this silent killer. This solid, well-organized site well fulfills its mission of educating the public.

Medical College of Wisconsin HealthLINK
www.healthlink.mcw.edu/high-blood-pressure

Source: 2
Navigation: 3
Interactivity: 1
Overall: 2

This site belongs to the Medical College of Wisconsin, and it's designed with patients in mind. The home page is simply organized, which allows you to access information without much hassle. You can read summaries from the latest research journals or find out what blood pressure news is making headlines. The site is all about information. Learn why it might be important to hold the salt!

MEDLINEplus on High Blood Pressure
www.nlm.nih.gov/medlineplus/highbloodpressure.html

Source: 3
Navigation: 3
Interactivity: 1
Overall: 3

The National Library of Medicine provides information from a variety of excellent sources on blood pressure. You'll be treated to information from the country's most reputable organizations and websites. Get the basics on high blood pressure or find out about clinical trials that are testing new medications. This is a great hub for hypertension information. Come here, and start on your way to finding reliable blood pressure info.

National Heart, Lung, and Blood Institute: Cardiovascular
   Information
www.nhlbi.nih.gov/health/public/heart

Source: 3
Navigation: 3
Interactivity: 2
Overall: 3

If you're looking for a variety of hypertension-related information, this could be the site for you. You can learn about the spe-
cially recommended DASH (Dietary Approaches to Stop
Hypertension) diet to help lower your blood pressure or find
out about the issue of hypertension in pregnancy. There is a link
to an interactive site that can help you lower your blood pressure and access to important information about cholesterol.
This site has something for everyone. Take your time to read,
note the prevention tips, and keep the old ticker healthy.

National Heart, Lung, and Blood Institute: Your Guide
   to Lowering High Blood Pressure
www.nhlbi.nih.gov/hbp

Source: 3
Navigation: 3
Interactivity: 2
Overall: 3

This site is one of the best interactive blood pressure sites on
the Net. It's part of the National Heart, Lung, and Blood Institute and provides information ranging from blood pressure
medications to prevention tips. The site is easy to navigate, and
the information is comprehensive. If you or a loved one has
high blood pressure, this site would be a great start on your
quest to bring those numbers down into the normal range.

HIV/AIDS

AIDS Clinical Trials Information Service
www.actis.org

Source: 3
Navigation: 3
Interactivity: 2
Overall: 3

This site is provided as a service by the U.S. Department of Health and Human Services. The primary aim of the site is to provide information on clinical trials that you or a loved one might be interested in joining. The site is extremely easy to navigate, and the information is written specifically for the public. Find drug, vaccine, or clinical trial information, or click on the links to other Net resources. This site also provides pages for those who speak Spanish. This is the best resource on the Net for finding a clinical trial.

AIDS.ORG
www.aids.org

Source: 2
Navigation: 3
Interactivity: 3
Overall: 3

This site is the epitome of one-stop HIV/AIDS information shopping. The site is easy to navigate because it's been organized so well. You'll find everything from the basics to the latest treatment news. Its community section is a great place to read and participate in discussion forums as well as chat online with others sharing similar concerns. There are a bookstore and links to other excellent Net resources. Stop by, you won't be disappointed.

AIDS Treatment Information Service
www.hivatis.org/trtgdlns.html

Source: 2
Navigation: 3
Interactivity: 2
Overall: 2

This site, a project of the U.S. Department of Health and Human Services, is cosponsored by several leading research institutions. It's specifically designed to bring you the latest in treatment recommendations. The information provided on this site draws from many of the leading governmental scientific institutes and organizations. The site is easy to navigate, and you don't need a science degree to understand its contents.

The Body: An AIDS and HIV Information Resource
www.thebody.com

Source: 2
Navigation: 3
Interactivity: 2
Overall: 2

This site belongs to an organization seeking to increase communication between doctors and researchers and the general public. Its advisory board includes many HIV/AIDS experts. The site covers the full range of information and is organized in a way that is easy to understand. You'll find everything from the basics on AIDS and prevention tips to understanding and possibly simplifying treatments. This site covers so many aspects of the disease that it's likely that most, if not all, of your questions will be answered.

Centers for Disease Control and Prevention on
    HIV/AIDS
www.cdc.gov/hiv/pubs/facts.htm

Source: 3
Navigation: 2
Interactivity: 1
Overall: 3

The Centers for Disease Control and Prevention is the country's epicenter of statistical and clinically relevant information on most of our infectious diseases. This is its métier, and it's not surprising that its website reflects that fact. You will find information ranging from the number of new HIV cases diagnosed each year to ways of preventing the disease. If you want HIV/AIDS information, this is a site you must stop by and learn from. There's so much here that you must take your time and absorb its riches like a sponge.

Gay Men's Health Crisis
www.gmhc.org

Source: 2
Navigation: 3
Interactivity: 3
Overall: 3

The Gay Men's Health Crisis in New York City was one of the first organizations in the world to take on the HIV/AIDS issue back in the early 1980s. Since then it's been a leader in educating and raising awareness about the disease and its devastating effects. The website stays true to the mission, providing excellent information about HIV and what it means to live with it. You can find out about the latest treatments and read headlines from journals around the world. This site will teach you not only about HIV but also what it means to be positive.

Harvard AIDS Institute
www.aids.harvard.edu

Source: 3
Navigation: 3
Interactivity: 1
Overall: 2

The Harvard AIDS Institute is one of the world's leading HIV/AIDS research centers. This is not a site where you'll learn the basics of HIV/AIDS. Instead, come here to learn about the latest research or find out what's happening on the laboratory benches that one day might affect the treatment of this deadly virus. There is also a resources section that sends you to different credible sources for information on various aspects of the disease. This site is not for the beginner, but if you're looking for the latest research, do stop by.

The Journal of the American Medical Association
   HIV/AIDS Resource Center
www.ama-assn.org/special/hiv/hivhome.htm

Source: 3
Navigation: 3
Interactivity: 1
Overall: 3

The Journal of the American Medical Association is one of the world's most respected journals. It's the publication of the largest doctors' organization in the country, the American Medical Association. With all of its resources, both financial and scientific, one would expect its site to be of equally high quality. The site is easy to navigate, and the content isn't too difficult to digest, even for a beginner. Read in-depth news reports, search millions of articles, or read about treatment guidelines. The site even provides a review of what the AMA considers to be some of the best HIV/AIDS Internet sites. This is a great place to start your search for HIV/AIDS information.

National Institute of Allergy and Infectious Diseases on the HIV-AIDS Connection
www.niaid.nih.gov/spotlight/hiv00

Source: 3
Navigation: 3
Interactivity: 1
Overall: 3

The NIAID is the U.S. research and educational home for infectious diseases. This site draws on one of the most extensive research databases in the world and opens it up to you in a way that's easy to navigate and a writing style you can understand. You'll find a full range of information on this site, and the majority of it will be what you're searching for: read fact sheets, learn about the latest presentations at the World AIDS Conference, or digest the latest treatment guidelines. The smart money says that what you're looking for can be found on this site or one of its links to other Net resources.

National Library of Medicine: Specialized Information Services
http://sis.nlm.nih.gov/hiv.cfm

Source: 3
Navigation: 3
Interactivity: 2
Overall: 3

This is the site of the largest electronic medical library on the planet, the National Library of Medicine. Here you'll find all the information you could ever want to know about the virus and advanced AIDS. The site is a breeze to navigate, and the links are extremely helpful and specific. It helps that the home page is so well organized that you don't have to fish around for information. You can read the latest news or learn about the most recent treatment guidelines with just a click. This is one of the Web's best hubs for HIV/AIDS info.

Hypertension
See **High Blood Pressure (Hypertension)**.

Kidney Disease

American Association of Kidney Patients
www.aakp.org

Source: 2
Navigation: 3
Interactivity: 1
Overall: 2

This organization bills itself as the only national kidney organization directed by kidney patients for kidney patients. The site offers patients information through a patient plan that provides a comprehensive guide to kidney disease as patients progress in their treatment. You can also read articles from the magazine *RenalLife,* which gives you the latest news in kidney disease and allows you to read encouraging stories from other patients. The information on this site is reviewed by a medical board with flying credentials.

American Kidney Fund
http://216.248.130.102

Source: 2
Navigation: 3
Interactivity: 2
Overall: 2

This site belongs to one of the large national voluntary health organizations that provides direct financial assistance for the benefit of kidney patients. You can find plenty of kidney disease facts on several conditions as well as order informational brochures. Learn the ins and outs of insurance and read about a discount pharmaceutical program. If you need help to pay for dialysis treatments or a transplant, this site can provide valuable information. This is a unique, service-oriented site that puts together resources and delivers assistance.

Georgetown University Nephrology Division
www.georgetown.edu/departments/medicine/nephrology

Source: 2
Navigation: 2
Interactivity: 1
Overall: 1

This site is well organized and easy to navigate, and depending on what you're looking for it may well answer your needs. There is not much on the basics of kidney disease; the site doesn't contain a long list of FAQs or fact sheets that detail the specifics of each disease. However, the site is redeemed by an extensive list of message boards in which you're invited to participate and one of the best groups of links to other kidney websites. If you can't find the information you want on this site, it will link you to one that will deliver.

iKidney.com
www.ikidney.com

Source: 1
Navigation: 3
Interactivity: 3
Overall: 2

This is a cool-looking website that makes surfing for information fun and not a chore. While it's light on the hard-core basics of kidney disease, it offers a lot of other resources. The community section allows you to post kidney-related messages and read other people's message as well as ask an expert a question. You can also read the encouraging stories of other kidney patients. If you plan on traveling and might have need of a dialysis center, you can access a database of dialysis centers throughout the United States. Don't leave without copying some of the tasty kidney-health recipes.

MEDLINEplus on Kidney Diseases
www.nlm.nih.gov/medlineplus/
    kidneydiseasesgeneral.html

Source: 3
Navigation: 3
Interactivity: 2
Overall: 3

If you want information on kidney disease, you couldn't pick a better place to look than this site, which covers a broad spectrum of diseases. There are also links to the best organizations and kidney-related resources on the Web. The "Clinical Trials" link informs you of the ongoing government-sponsored trials on various kidney diseases. There's even a section on kidney disease statistics. If you need the facts on a particular kidney condition, you won't be let down.

National Institute of Diabetes & Digestive & Kidney
  Diseases
www.niddk.nih.gov

Source: 3
Navigation: 3
Interactivity: 1
Overall: 3

If you're looking for information on kidney disease, this is the
place to start and in some cases end your search. This is one of
only a few sites that contains a complete database on the various kidney-related diseases. The information is extremely accessible and written in a way that makes sense to the layperson.
The site is easy to navigate, and finding the information you
need couldn't be simpler. As on many government sites, there
isn't much in the way of interactivity, but the content is so comprehensive that I can't help but cast it as one of the best sites on
the Web.

National Kidney Foundation
www.kidney.org

Source: 2
Navigation: 3
Interactivity: 2
Overall: 2

This site belongs to one of the foremost kidney foundations in
the world. It provides information for both professionals and
consumers. You can learn all about kidney transplants, whether
you're a donor or recipient. You can also read the latest research
and news by clicking the "Electronic Kidney" link. The site's
content is quite thorough and easy to read, making it one of the
best places to learn about the organs that help you winkle.

NephrologyChannel
www.nephrologychannel.com

Source: 3
Navigation: 3
Interactivity: 3
Overall: 3

This is the ultimate in one-stop shopping for kidney information. You'll find plenty of information on a broad spectrum of diseases, many of which you've never heard of before. This site also has some of the best kidney chat rooms I've seen on the Net. You can chat with a professional or another patient. You can also read the latest news in kidney health. If you think you need a kidney doctor but don't know where to look for one, try the M.D. locator, which can help you find the nephrologist nearest you.

Nephron Information Center
www.nephron.com

Source: 3
Navigation: 3
Interactivity: 2
Overall: 3

If you visit this site at the beginning of your search, you might never leave it. It provides almost anything you can think of related to kidney disease. There's a long list of hot kidney topics that brings you up-to-date on the latest kidney news. Visit the "Nephroquest" section, where you can read and post messages on a variety of kidney diseases. The site's database of dialysis centers will tell you which is the one nearest you. You can also read the pages in five other languages, including Spanish and French. The links are extensive and some of the most specific I've seen. This site is your total kidney package.

RENALNET: Kidney Information Clearinghouse
www.renalnet.org

Source: 3
Navigation: 2
Interactivity: 1
Overall: 2

This is the place to go for entry into the web of kidney disease information. The site contains an extremely comprehensive database and list of resources, whether you're in need of a kidney transplant or want to find out what "glomerulonephritis" means. By clicking on the "Conference Room" link on www.renalnet.org/renalnet/features/about.cfm, you can joint a chat on kidney disease. There are numerous chat rooms available for everyone from administrators to patients. If you're looking for a home base for Net information on kidney disease, welcome!

Liver/Cirrhosis

American Liver Foundation
www.liverfoundation.org

Source: 3
Navigation: 3
Interactivity: 3
Overall: 3

This can definitely be the site where you both begin your education and end your searches on liver disorders. It is comprehensive and easy to navigate, covering general topics and branching into specific liver disorders. It is particularly enjoyable to read the section of stories of those with liver disorders—the result of efforts on the part of the site to promote a sense of community among those who suffer from liver problems. Finally, its links to support groups are solid, and for those looking for further assistance, these should be taken into account as well.

Columbia University on Liver Diseases
www.cpmcnet.columbia.edu/dept/gi/disliv.html

Source: 2
Credibility: 3
Interactivity: 1
Overall: 2

Here is a very comprehensive, detailed, and trustworthy site that directs you to other sites based on the disorder you want to learn about. The sources are extremely credible, and the information provided is definitely thorough. The site may look a bit intimidating at first because of its monotonous appearance and often complex writing, and it needs to be updated more frequently, yet it is an excellent source of general liver information.

Loyola University Health System
www.luhs.org/health/topics/liver

Source: 3
Navigation: 3
Interactivity: 1
Overall: 2

This is a very easy to navigate site that provides credible information on the liver and its associated disorders. It is a great educational site, a place to learn about liver function, symptoms of disorders, and possible treatments. In general, it is a place anyone seeking general information on the liver and its conditions should visit.

MEDLINEplus on Cirrhosis
www.nlm.nih.gov/medlineplus/cirrhosis.html

Source: 3
Navigation: 2
Interactivity: 1
Overall: 2

This compilation site, made up of many great links, makes the search for liver information easier on you, the patient, by providing you with credible, easy-to-find information. Though the site may seem slightly intimidating at first, it is nice to know that it has done some of the research for you and may be able to send you on the right path to find the information you're looking for.

The PBC Foundation
www.nhtech.demon.co.uk/pbc

Source: 2
Navigation: 3
Interactivity: 1
Overall: 2

Here is a site primarily designed for cirrhosis sufferers; a good place to begin within this site is with its simplified explanation of the liver and how it works. It is particularly strong in addressing primary biliary cirrhosis (PBC) and the information is thorough as well as containing a good segment on how doctors should treat PBC sufferers, something all patients would be well served by reading as well. Finally, it addresses the patient in various ways by offering tips, the best of which is definitely its "how to deal with itching" advice.

PBC Patient Support Network
www.superaje.com/~pbc

Source: 1
Navigation: 3
Interactivity: 3
Overall: 2

This site provides a brief overview of PBC with accompanying facts, but it is not wise to come here as your source for background and general information. Instead, the strength of this site is its strong discussion forum, which is dedicated to helping sufferers of PBC and their family members support each other. The posts are thoughtfully written and responses are almost always posted, making it an active forum.

University of Chicago Liver Study Unit
http://gi.bsd.uchicago.edu/diseases/liverdisease/
    liverdisease.html

Source: 3
Navigation: 3
Interactivity: 1
Overall: 2

This is a great site on which to begin a search about liver disorders, as it provides solid information on the liver itself along with easy access to information regarding the various liver disorders. The information is clearly presented, and the site is well organized. There's something here for all of us to learn.

Lyme Disease

ACP-ASIM Online: Initiative on Lyme Disease
www.acponline.org/lyme/patient

Source: 3
Credibility: 3
Interactivity: 1
Overall: 1

This is an extremely easy-to-use site. You will not find the slightest problem with locating information, though the degree of detail is not as strong as I would like. It is the perfect site, however, for those looking for quick answers to broad questions about Lyme disease. It is highly credible and run by a staff made up mainly of physicians.

American Lyme Disease Foundation, Inc.
www.aldf.com

Source: 3
Navigation: 2
Interactivity: 1
Overall: 2

This site is very easy to get through, and you will not be disappointed with the information supplied. It will give you a good understanding of Lyme disease, with particularly interesting facts such as the distribution of Lyme disease by state. The site, however, does need to be updated more frequently, since at the date of this writing it has been stagnant for some time.

Ask NOAH About: Lyme Disease
www.noah-health.org/english/illness/lyme/lyme.html

Source: 3
Navigation: 1
Interactivity: 2
Overall: 2

A broad range of categories is presented on this site, each one describing different facets of the disease as well as target groups. The opening page is long and may be a bit confusing at first since it is very monotonous in the way it is arranged. However, if you can get past that, the facts are detailed and credible and there are enormous amounts of information. In addition, there are valuable links to discussion forums so that you can discuss your problems with others.

Centers for Disease Control and Prevention of Lyme
   Disease
www.cdc.gov/ncidad/dvbid/lymeinfo.htm

Source: 3
Credibility: 3
Interactivity: 1
Overall: 3

At first glance you can tell that this site is one extremely well organized location, put together by people who know what they are doing. It has loads of credible information, which it has organized into categories ranging from history to diagnosis to prevention and control. I particularly enjoyed the precision with which it describes the process of removing a tick. Finally, seeing such a strong FAQs section, it is easy to tell that this is a site on which many of your questions can and will be answered.

Lyme Disease Foundation
www.lyme.org

Source: 3
Navigation: 2
Interactivity: 2
Overall: 2

The winner of an award from the National Institutes of Health, this site provides information on Lyme disease from all angles, from history to treatment, and provides high-quality pictures of ticks and symptoms. Perhaps the most enjoyable section of this site are the pages of stories of those who have had to deal with Lyme disease, fostering a feeling of camaraderie with those with the illness that other sites do not.

Lyme Disease Network
www.lymenet.org

Source: 2
Credibility: 3
Interactivity: 3
Overall: 2

If you're looking for interaction, discussions, and Web forums, this is an excellent place to visit. The message boards are active, and the posts are very informative. The site's strength is its pictures of ticks and early symptoms worth noting, but if your prime concern is gathering information, this is not the first place to visit as the forums are the best part.

MEDLINEplus on Lyme Disease
www.nlm.nih.gov/medlineplus/lymedisease.html

Source: 3
Navigation: 2

Interactivity: 1
Overall: 2

Here is a potpourri of information, including a collection of the National Institutes of Health's own information, such as pictures and facts, as well as links to the best features of other Lyme disease sites. It is a great place to visit if you want to visit only one site that hand-selects articles from other top-notch sites. It is exceptionally well organized, separating age groups in terms of targeting. The site might initially be intimidating for some, but be encouraged—your efforts to get past your first impression will be rewarded.

University of Connecticut: Lyme Disease Education
www.ucc.uconn.edu/~wwwlyme

Source: 3
Navigation: 3
Interactivity: 3
Overall: 3

This is a very patient-friendly site, one that not only is easy to use but presents well-documented information. One of its greatest strengths is its educational games, which are fun and interactive, and, when coupled with its presentation format, make it a great site for both youths and adults.

Menopause

American College of Obstetricians and Gynecologists
www.acog.org

Source: 3
Navigation: 3

Interactivity: 1
Overall: 3

Here's a good site to gather peer-reviewed information on menopause. Information is organized from introductory to advanced/professional research. Some of the advanced or professional articles may be difficult reading, and you'll have to work around some advertising, but you'll find reputable, solid information if you persist. A wide range of topics is discussed from choosing the best form of hormone replacement to some nontraditional ways to relieve those annoying hot flashes.

The Foundation for Better Health Care on Menopause
www.fbhc.org/patients/betterhealth/menopause/
    home.html

Source: 3
Navigation: 1
Interactivity: 1
Overall: 2

This site is sponsored by a not-for-profit educational organization that is accredited by the Accreditation Council for Continuing Medical Education. The information is easy to read, well organized, and a good reference for women facing menopause. You'll find the information written for the layperson, and almost all of the relevant topics are well covered. You can get a better understanding of what progesterone and estrogen do to the body and the health changes you can expect after menopause. If you want to know more, check out the FAQs and read till you're content.

MayoClinic.com on Menopause
www.mayoclinic.com/home?id=DS00119

Source: 3
Navigation: 3
Interactivity: 1
Overall: 3

Start your search on menopause here. It is well organized and easy to navigate. The information is also easy to read and understand. The site is regularly reviewed and updated by Mayo Clinic researchers and physicians, thus providing it with authoritative source material.

Menopause Online
www.menopauseonline.com

Source: 2
Navigation: 2
Interactivity: 1
Overall: 1

If you're looking for information on the alternative and complementary treatments women are using to treat their menopausal symptoms, this is a site you must visit. Its credibility is backed by a group of professionals who handle the editing chores. To lighten the mood, you can read some of the comic relief, and for interaction, you can read and post to the bulletin board. Another plus is free MEDLINEplus search access.

National Women's Health Resource Center
www.healthywomen.org

Source: 3
Navigation: 3

Interactivity: 1
Overall: 3

This site is well organized and easy to navigate. Each topic contains references, and all content is reviewed by medical professionals. The site only uses peer-reviewed, reputable journals, as well as books generally not more than one to two years old, published by experts. It is concise, easy to understand, and accurate. You'll find important information about many of the menopausal symptoms and gain insight into the heavily debated hormone replacement therapy and why it may or may not be right for you.

North American Menopause Society
www.menopause.org

Source: 2
Navigation: 3
Interactivity: 1
Overall: 2

This site contains referral lists, basic facts, statistics, and a useful, informative, downloadable booklet. Suggested readings, terms, various therapies, and additional resources are also included and very useful. You'll find important information about symptoms and how best to deal with them.

Planned Parenthood on Menopause
www.plannedparenthood.org/womenshealth/
    menopause.htm

Source: 3
Navigation: 2
Interactivity: 1
Overall: 2

The information on this site is presented in an easy-to-read, understandable format. It also contains additional references and resources. This is a good reference site to learn about symptoms, treatment, and coping mechanisms. You'll also find plenty of information about both traditional and alternative treatments.

Women's Health Interactive on Midlife Health
www.womens-health.com/health_center/midlife

Source: 2
Navigation: 3
Interactivity: 2
Overall: 2

This site is well organized and easy to navigate. It contains self-assessments and comprehensive, clear information. It also has really good graphics and a pleasing design. There is excellent interaction through discussion forums, and you can browse the health centers to find everything involving reproductive health as well as perimenopausal and menopausal issues. Menstrual disorders are discussed, and it's all laid out in an easy-to-use format. Check out the quality-of-midlife study in the research center.

Mental Health

Center for Mental Health Services Knowledge
    Exchange Network
www.mentalhealth.org

Source: 2
Navigation: 3

Interactivity: 1
Overall: 2

This site contains extensive information including fact sheets, news articles, networking, discrimination and rights, and the stigma associated with mental illness. There's something here for everyone from professionals to parents of children with mental illness. If you can't find what you're looking for, try the links. For those who speak Spanish, there are pages here for you also.

Mental Help Net
www.mentalhelp.net

Source: 2
Navigation: 2
Interactivity: 2
Overall: 2

Go to this site to learn about specific mental disorders and treatments; there are community message boards, a mental health glossary of terms, some humor, and even an online therapist (just for fun).

National Alliance for the Mentally Ill
www.nami.org

Source: 1
Navigation: 3
Interactivity: 1
Overall: 1

This site is a well-organized resource for people afflicted with mental illness and their family members. It is easy to navigate and covers the spectrum of mental illness and support resources. You'll find fact sheets on the general topic of mental illness as well as information regarding mental illness in children and adolescents. Check the pressroom and get the recent headlines or read the latest advocacy issues. There's something here for everyone.

National Institute of Mental Health
www.nimh.nih.gov

Source: 3
Navigation: 2
Interactivity: 1
Overall: 3

This site contains a wealth of information on a variety of mental illnesses, including child and adolescent mental health issues. You'll find the site easy to navigate and orderly in its presentation. Look for information on clinical trials and a link to MEDLINEplus to search for peer-reviewed full-text journal articles.

National Mental Health Association
www.nmha.org

Source: 2
Navigation: 3
Interactivity: 2
Overall: 2

This not-for-profit organization site has an excellent search engine that takes you quickly to the site's referral services, screening tests, e-alerts, and chat opportunities. Concise fact sheets that are easily understood are also provided. This is a well-rounded informational site.

National Mental Health Consumers' Self-Help
   Clearinghouse
www.mhselfhelp.org

Source: 1
Navigation: 3
Interactivity: 1
Overall: 1

This is a consumer-run national technical assistance center that includes information in Spanish. The site contains multiple tools and resources to empower individuals in making choices about their mental health. This site is less about information and more about connecting people to services. Find out about political issues related to mental health or self-help groups. You can also read the latest in mental health news by clicking on the updates and information.

Myaligic Encephalmyelitis
(See **Chronic Fatigue Syndrome.**)

Nutrition

American Dietetic Association
www.eatright.org

Source: 3
Navigation: 3
Interactivity: 2
Overall: 3

If you want to find information about nutrition and healthy eating, this should be your first stop. Here you'll find extensive nu-

tritional fact sheets as well as an illustration of the food pyramid. Find out how calcium can help prevent osteoporosis. You'll
also be given access to excerpts from the association's food and
nutrition guide. This site can help make eating healthy fun.

Food and Nutrition Information Center
www.nalusda.gov/fnic

Source: 3
Navigation: 3
Interactivity: 2
Overall: 3

This is undoubtedly one of the best nutritional sites on the Net.
You can find out almost anything you need to know—if not on
this site, then through one of its many excellent links to other
great sources of information. You can read about the composi-
tion of the food you eat, then check out the dietary guidelines.
Want more? Look at the food pyramid to make sure you're eating those five servings of fruits and vegetables a day. You'll get
information on everything from school meals to food safety.
This could be the only site you'll ever need to log on to when
searching for nutrition information.

MayoClinic.com Food & Nutrition Center
www.mayoclinic.com/home?id=4.1.5

Source: 3
Navigation: 3
Interactivity: 2
Overall: 3

One of the most respected medical centers in the world, the
Mayo Clinic, has built a food and nutrition site that lives up to
the institution's vast reputation. The home page is neatly orga-

nized into different features. You can learn how to eat well and healthily and then click on another feature to discover the connection between food and health. Have questions about supplements? Those answers are there for you, as are tips to keep those extra pounds off of your waistline. It's easy to read, comprehensive, and extremely credible—what more can you ask for in a website?

MEDLINEplus on Nutrition
www.nlm.nih.gov/medlineplus/nutrition.html

Source: 3
Navigation: 3
Interactivity: 1
Overall: 3

There are plenty of excellent nutrition sites on the Web, but this one is exceptional. Here, you'll find answers to specific questions, such as how to change your eating habits and be more physically active. The beauty of this site, however, is that it draws its information from other sites that are the best in the business. If you're looking for a nutrition hub that can guide you to a wide array of Internet nutrition sources, you've found the spot.

National Dairy Council
www.nationaldairycouncil.org

Source: 2
Navigation: 2
Interactivity: 1
Overall: 2

If your questions involve dairy products, don't look any further. You'll find out more about cheese, milk, and yogurt than you ever imagined. Are you lactose-intolerant and experiencing difficulty digesting dairy products? Maybe you suffer from high blood pressure and need a low-salt diet? This site gives you tips on nutrients and then offers links to other websites that can also be of assistance. Got milk? Get this website.

Nutri-Facts.com
www.nutri-facts.com

Source: 2
Navigation: 3
Interactivity: 3
Overall: 3

Have you ever wanted to calculate your body mass index (BMI)? Better still, how many calories are in that big piece of apple pie? This website can give you answers to both those questions and more. You can read and post messages on the bulletin board or do searches on different foods to find out more about their nutritional content. Are you a fast-food junkie? Find out what you're really putting into your body. This site contains important information about what we like to eat and what we should eat. Stop here, and you might think twice about that large order of fries.

NutritionResource.com
www.nutritionresource.com

Source: 3
Navigation: 3
Interactivity: 2
Overall: 3

This website is managed by a team of registered dieticians who are experts on foods and what they provide to our bodies. It's a site that's easy to navigate, and the information is written for everyone to understand. You'll be able to read about everything from low-carbohydrate diets to eating plans for vegetarian athletes. If you have a couple of questions, run them by a dietician during the discussion forum. It's difficult to imagine that there are many questions about nutrition that this site or its links can't answer.

Tufts Nutrition Navigator
www.navigator.tufts.edu

Source: 3
Navigation: 3
Interactivity: 2
Overall: 3

This is by far my favorite all-around health site on the Web. It is neatly divided into different sections, and the design is active without being too busy. You can find so much information that you may never need to leave. Get the skinny on hot topics or read about special dietary needs for certain body types. Not visiting this site is like going to Paris for the first time and not going to the top of the Eiffel Tower.

U.S. Food and Drug Administration Center for Food
    Safety and Applied Nutrition
www.cfsan.fda.gov

Source: 2
Navigation: 3
Interactivity: 1
Overall: 2

If you have questions regarding food safety or dietary supplements, this is the site to visit. The FDA, the major regulator of food products, has extensive information on these topics. The writing can be dense at times, but the information is the best you'll find. You can learn about foodborne illnesses, canned foods, and food additives. If you don't mind sifting through extra pages to get to the information you want, you can find some gems.

Obesity/Weight Control

American Dietetic Association
www.eatright.org

Source: 3
Navigation: 3
Interactivity: 2
Overall: 2

This association of food experts has put together a website for the public and health professionals. The information accessible by the public is extremely informative and easy to read. You can read excerpts from the book *Dieting for Dummies,* which covers a broad range of topics from changing your diet attitude to the top ten myths of dieting. Where better to get information about weight management than the place that knows every morsel about the contents of our food?

American Heart Association
www.americanheart.org

Source: 3
Navigation: 3
Interactivity: 1
Overall: 3

Why go to a heart association's website for weight management information? Answer: the American Heart Association has done tremendous work on nutrition and exercise programs that are healthy not only for your heart but for your overall health. Just enter the "Family Health" section, where you can click on the exercise or nutrition links. Then watch those pounds fall off as you begin taking advantage of the healthy weight reduction tips.

American Obesity Association
www.obesity.org

Source: 3
Navigation: 3
Interactivity: 1
Overall: 3

If you want information on obesity and what it may be doing to your health, you've found an excellent site. The content is extremely well written, thorough, and accessible. Navigating the site is effortless, and you can read extensively about all of the issues surrounding obesity and its negative health implications. Do you want to learn more about obesity surgery? There is an information cluster that will tell you all about it. This is an excellent site to learn how to burn off those extra calories.

CBS HealthWatch on Weight Management
www.cbshealthwatch.medscape.com/
    weightmanagementcenter

Source: 2
Navigation: 3
Interactivity: 3
Overall: 2

So you're tired of yo-yo dieting and those gimmick diets that promise to help you lose half of yourself overnight. Well, this is a place to begin your new quest for a meaner and leaner body. The information is well organized and easy to read, and the tips are reasonable. There are also excellent interactive tools, such as a message board that allows you to read and post information about your weight loss experience. Come here for reality, not gimmicks.

Medscape on Weight Management
www.medscape.com/Medscape/features/ResourceCenter/
    obesity/public/RC-index-obesity.html

Source: 2
Navigation: 2
Interactivity: 3
Overall: 2

It's difficult to find many sites that are honest about weight loss and the science behind what it takes to shed those extra pounds. Medscape, one of the most credible medical information sources on the Net, deals with weight loss information as it does everything else: cautiously, thoroughly, and with credibility. The information here will enlighten you about the epidemic of obesity and its implications for your health. The site is divided into sections that make it easy for you to navigate and find the information you need. After digesting all of the information offered here, exercise the links and connect to other important weight management sites on the Net.

National Heart, Lung, and Blood Institute on Weight
www.nhlbi.nih.gov/health/public/heart/obesity/lose_wt

Source: 3
Navigation: 3

Interactivity: 2
Overall: 3

This is a well-organized site that has areas sectioned off for patients and one for health professionals. The site allows you to assess your risk of developing heart disease by calculating your BMI (body mass index) and looking for other risk factors such as smoking. There aren't any gimmicks here, just solid information about nutrition and weight management and what everyone needs to know about how what goes into your mouth can end up on your waistline.

National Institute of Diabetes & Digestive & Kidney
    Diseases on Nutrition
www.niddk.nih.gov/health/nutrit/nutrit.htm

Source: 3
Navigation: 3
Interactivity: 1
Overall: 3

This site has top-drawer credibility and excellent, easy-to-follow information on eating disorders, obesity in children and teenagers, and health concerns of various kinds of dieting. The site includes a section on health issues related to very-low-calorie and fad diets. The material is presented as a table of contents, so it is easy to find specific answers to questions.

North American Association for the Study of Obesity
www.naaso.org

Source: 3
Navigation: 3
Interactivity: 1
Overall: 1

Consult this website if you want the real deal on the latest re-search and headlines regarding obesity. Consider this more of an information site and less of an interactive one where you work on a program to lose weight. The content is thorough and makes for an interesting read even for those who might not nec-essarily be interested in losing weight. You won't find links to other sites, but what you get here will go a long way in satisfy-ing your hunger for weight management news.

Partnership for Healthy Weight Management
www.consumer.gov/weightloss

Source: 2
Navigation: 3
Interactivity: 1
Overall: 2

This is a site that gives you the truth about dieting and weight management. It's the brainchild of a coalition of representa-tives from science, academia, the health care profession, gov-ernment, commercial enterprises, and organizations whose mission is to promote sound strategies for achieving and main-taining healthy weight. The information is direct and brutally honest, yet still encouraging. If you want to prepare yourself mentally to control your weight, start here!

Shape Up America!
www.shapeup.org

Source: 3
Navigation: 2
Interactivity: 3
Overall: 3

Dr. C. Everett Koop, former U.S. surgeon general, was one of the founders of this nationwide initiative to reduce obesity and increase the country's health. The goal of this site is to inform people of the benefits of physical exercise and good nutrition. The site is dedicated to consumers, so the information is easy to read and the site is easy to navigate. Make sure you visit the Body Fat Lab to find out if there's too much around your waistline and the effect this excess can have on your health. The measurement tools will teach you the various ways to measure your body fat and calculate that trendy weight measure, the BMI or body mass index.

Obstetrics and Gynecology
(Also see **Reproductive Health.**)

American College of Obstetricians and Gynecologists
www.acog.org

Source: 3
Navigation: 3
Interactivity: 1
Overall: 3

This is one of the premier sites for obstetrics and gynecologic issues. It has miles of information, and most important, you'll be able to understand it. It tackles more women's health problems than you ever dreamed existed. The site tells you what it has right on the home page, making it easy and fun to navigate. If this is your first stop for ob/gyn info, it could justifiably be your one and only.

MedNets on Obstetrics and Gynecology
www.mednets.com/obgynpat.htm

Source: 1
Navigation: 3
Interactivity: 1
Overall: 1

This site gives you information on a variety of issues ranging from pregnancy and menopause to cancer and bladder problems. The site is designed for easy navigation and quick learning. You can opt to use the patients' engine to search the site or try MEDLINEplus. Between the information the site offers and its external sources, your questions are sure to be answered.

OBGYN.net
www.obgyn.net

Source: 2
Navigation: 3
Interactivity: 2
Overall: 2

This site is a wonderful resource for those who are searching for ob/gyn information. The "Women's Pavilion" is the depot for issues ranging from pregnancy to endometriosis. It's written in a way consumers can understand, and you can navigate to other sources of information. The discussion forums are especially valuable and cover a wide range of topics from ultrasound to breast cancer. You'll find various articles written by medical professionals. This is a site that spans the globe of ob/gyn information.

Virtual Hospital on Obstetrics and Gynecology
www.vh.org/Patients/IHB/ObGyn.html

Source: 2
Navigation: 3
Interactivity: 1
Overall: 1

This site does three things: inform, inform, inform. There aren't any advertising distractions or solicitations, just links to a long list of female-related health issues. The information is written by professionals for patients, making it scientifically credible but consumer-friendly at the same time. Whether you're researching a common disease or one that's quite rare, you're likely to find your answers on this site.

Oral Health

American Dental Association
www.ada.org

Source: 3
Navigation: 3
Interactivity: 1
Overall: 3

The ultimate trustworthy source of information about oral health, this site can be the beginning, middle, and end of your search for knowledge. It goes from the general, such as tooth-brushing technique, to the specifics about different oral diseases. The site is comprehensive, extremely easy to use, and frequently updated. No site could make you feel more comfortable.

American Dental Hygienists' Association
www.adha.org

Source: 3
Navigation: 3
Interactivity: 1
Overall: 2

The American Dental Hygienists' Association has created a great site on which to begin your search for information about oral health, as it contains all sorts of information ranging from how to brush your teeth correctly to how to choose a dentist. It's well organized and easy to navigate, and it's a must visit for all those looking for quality general information.

Arizona Office of Oral Health: Oral Health Education
    Resources
www.hs.state.az.us/cfhs/ooh/edresources.htm

Source: 3
Navigation: 3
Interactivity: 1
Overall: 2

An easy-to-use site, this is a collection of quality links to other sites organized into categories in a user-friendly format. The links are definitely highly trustworthy and well organized. This should be the first site you visit, as it will guide you in the proper direction.

The Dental Consumer Advisor
www.toothinfo.com

Source: 2
Navigation: 3

Interactivity: 1
Overall: 2

The site is dedicated to educating you, the patient, and it succeeds in that endeavor. By disseminating general facts, teaching you terminology, and making you familiar with insurance—as well as the dental images you'll see—this site will make you a better-informed consumer. It is not a site where you'll find detailed information about any one area, but you'll definitely be better-rounded in your general understanding after reading its pages.

The Dental Site: Dental Resources for Patients
www.dentalsite.com/patients

Source: 2
Navigation: 2
Interactivity: 1
Overall: 1

You'll find general information here, mostly through links to other credible sites. The links are not as strong as those of other sites, but one particular link is interesting—it deals with the fear of going to a dentist and how to handle it.

National Center for Chronic Disease Prevention and
    Health Promotion: Oral Health Resources
www.cdc.gov/nccdphp/oh

Source: 2
Navigation: 3
Interactivity: 1
Overall: 1

Here is an extremely user-friendly educational site that provides general information in categories ranging from water fluoridation to cancer to cutting-edge research. The research section needs to be updated more frequently to be fully reliable, but this is nonetheless a good place to begin researching general questions about symptoms and basic treatments.

National Institute of Dental and Craniofacial Research
www.nidr.nih.gov

Source: 3
Navigation: 2
Interactivity: 1
Overall: 2

The site contains a wide variety of oral health information from healthy baby mouths to smart snacking. It is easy to use and well organized, and it takes you step by step through whatever category of oral health you are searching, to ease your anxiety with sound research. It is a site where both basic information and extensive research can be found.

Oral Health America
www.oralhealthamerica.org

Source: 3
Navigation: 2
Interactivity: 1
Overall: 1

Much of this site, which is not generally difficult to navigate, leads to more articles about the foundation itself. However, once you get to the information pages the high quality of the material is obvious. Of particular interest to me were the individual grades given in various subjects such as fluoridation and health care in all fifty states. There are also various high-quality articles covering topics from general oral health facts to dental insurance.

ParentsPlace.com: Dentist
www.parentsplace.com/expert/dentist

Source: 3
Navigation: 3
Interactivity: 2
Overall: 2

The site features a wide array of questions in all areas of oral health asked of an expert dentist and professor. The questions cover many common concerns you may have had at some point, arranged in categories for easy access. It is not necessarily the best place to gain general knowledge, but for specific concerns it may be very helpful.

Osteoporosis

American Academy of Orthopaedic Surgeons
http://orthoinfo.aaos.org

Source: 3
Navigation: 3
Interactivity: 1
Overall: 1

This site is run by doctors who treat the fractures that can develop as a result of osteoporosis. If they don't know about this disease, who does? Here you'll find tons of information on everything from ways to prevent osteoporosis nutritionally to tips on decreasing your risk for fractures. There aren't any links to other sites, which would make it more user-friendly, but the content is especially created for consumers and written in a style that helps you understand without any hassle.

Colorado HealthSite
www.coloradohealthnet.org

Source: 2
Navigation: 3
Interactivity: 3
Overall: 3

This site will provide you with basic information on osteoporosis that doesn't take a science degree to comprehend. There are a library and an internal search engine that turn up information on demand. You can also ask an expert a question or sign up with the "Pen Pals" service and discuss your condition and experience with someone else. Check out the cool banner on the top of the page that gives you flashes on breaking osteoporosis news.

EndocrineWeb.com: The Osteoporosis Center
www.endocrineweb.com/osteoporosis

Source: 3
Navigation: 3
Interactivity: 3
Overall: 3

What better place to find information about osteoporosis than a site that specializes in endocrinology? This site offers a complete guide to osteoporosis, covering a vast array of topics and presenting the information in an easy-to-read format. Navigation isn't a hurdle with this site, as the links are laid out clearly and in an orderly fashion. I'm not too excited about the product hawking at the bottom of the page, but it's out of the way and won't interrupt your search. This site will quench your thirst for osteoporosis information.

HeliosHealth.com on Osteoporosis
www.helioshealth.com/osteoporosis

Source: 2
Navigation: 3
Interactivity: 2
Overall: 2

This site provides accurate, current information about osteoporosis and its treatments. You'll find the latest headlines regarding this debilitating and unnecessary medical condition. You can also join a chat room and talk to others who have battled the disease. Before leaving, take a look at the section on the importance of vitamin D and calcium and what they do to preserve our bones.

International Osteoporosis Foundation
www.osteofound.org

Source: 3
Navigation: 2
Interactivity: 1
Overall: 2

This is another excellent source for osteoporosis information. Beyond reading the basics about osteoporosis, you can link up to osteoporosis societies and resources around the globe. You can also read interesting patient accounts about battles with osteoporosis and what others have done to try to prevent it from destroying their lives. Feel free to share your story and read other stories as they come in from all parts of the world. You can also read past articles and clinical findings, all in an effort to keep your bones strong.

National Institutes of Health on Osteoporosis and
    Related Bone Diseases
www.osteo.org

Source: 3
Navigation: 3
Interactivity: 2
Overall: 3

The National Institutes of Health is one of the world's leading
scientific/medical clinical and research systems. It's no surprise
that its websites are some of the best you can find on the Net.
This site is no exception, providing thorough, easy-to-read information that covers osteoporosis from A to Z. You can also
make use of the extensive list of links to other Net resources.
While you're here, you can read about other bone diseases.
Those who speak only Spanish, do not be dismayed—there are
pages of information in Spanish also. This is one of the most informative osteoporosis sites on the Web.

National Osteoporosis Foundation
www.nof.org

Source: 3
Navigation: 3
Interactivity: 3
Overall: 3

This must be your first stop when cruising the Net for osteoporosis information. This site has everything you can imagine.
The information is reliable, current, and easy to read. The site
is a navigation cinch because everything is laid out openly and
neatly. You might never want to leave the site because it's so
fulfilling, especially with its support groups and links to finding
a doctor. It's difficult to imagine that you'll need to look at
many other sites after visiting this one.

National Ostoporosis Society
www.nos.org.uk

Source: 3
Navigation: 3
Interactivity: 1
Overall: 2

Osteoporosis isn't just an American disease, it's a worldwide problem. This British site, of the National Osteoporosis Society, gives us a look at the disease across the Atlantic. Some of the statistics might be different, but the basics are the same. This site contains excellent information on prevention, diagnosis, and treatment. The personal profiles will better help you understand how global and dangerous a disease it is, and the links will send you to all corners of the world for the best osteoporosis information available.

Osteoporosis and Bone Physiology
http://courses.washington.edu/bonephys

Source: 2
Navigation: 3
Interactivity: 1
Overall: 2

This site doesn't have many interactive tools, but it is certainly content-heavy, full of excellent information that explains exactly what osteoporosis is and why some of us develop it. This is an educational site, so the advertisements are minimal and the learning possibilities are maximized. There's a kids' corner that reviews bone biology, and it's just as good for adults as kids. There aren't any links to other websites, but if you read all of the pages on this site, you might not need another source. Come here to really learn the facts about osteoporosis.

Osteoporosis Society of Canada
www.osteoporosis.ca

Source: 3
Navigation: 3
Interactivity: 1
Overall: 2

Welcome to the home of the Osteoporosis Society of Canada. This is a well-organized site that makes searching for osteoporosis information easy. It's written with you, the consumer, in mind, and it gives you the info you need—from a clear definition of osteoporosis to important tips on prevention and treatment. Once you've gotten your fill of information, travel the links to other Net sources. Naturally, these pages are available in French also.

Pain Management

American Academy of Pain Management
www.aapainmanage.org

Source: 3
Navigation: 2
Interactivity: 3
Overall: 2

This is a great place to begin, especially if you are looking for physicians. Although definitions of pain management are given, the site is not nearly as specific as it should be with regard to various kinds of pain. The best part of this site is definitely its forum, which is important and appears to be the most heavily trafficked part of the site.

New York University: Pain Management Center
www.med.nyu.edu/PainManagement

Source: 2
Navigation: 3
Interactivity: 1
Overall: 2

This is a very credible site, but not one that is easy to read once you get into the category of pain management you have looked up. However, if you do read through it all, you will find the information to be very thorough and you will feel that you understand what is going on in your body.

Pain.com
www.pain.com

Source: 2
Navigation: 3
Interactivity: 3
Overall: 3

Here is a strong, very easy to use site, with a broad range of pain categories and ideas of how to deal with them presented in the form of articles about everything from migraines to anesthesia. Updates occur daily here, with new articles appearing from journals. The site is friendly to the user and an emphasis is also placed on interaction.

PainLink
www.edc.org/PainLink

Source: 3
Navigation: 2
Interactivity: 2
Overall: 2

This is definitely not the easiest site to navigate, as a certain amount of time and specificity is required from you, but the results will be well worth it if you choose to look around. Especially useful is the section on pain in distinct populations, which can direct you anywhere from pain management in nursing homes to the special concerns of women and those with terminal illnesses.

Pain Management Online
www.painmngt.com

Source: 3
Navigation: 2
Interactivity: 1
Overall: 2

This site is particularly strong in the area of headaches. The information is very detail-oriented and at times seems to be geared to professionals. Nonetheless, some of the pain management issues that are discussed on a high level may be useful if you couple your reading with consulting a physician or if you are searching for very advanced material. There is a wide array of categories, and you'll find details about all different kinds of pain and suffering.

Pain Net
www.painnet.com

Source: 2
Navigation: 2
Interactivity: 1
Overall: 2

The site starts with general information, but if you desire more, through careful selection you can find some outstandingly thorough information on some areas of pain management. It would be nice if there were more categories, but the site covers the general areas very well.

Parkinson's Disease

About.com on Parkinson's Disease Drugs
and Treatments
www.pharmacology.about.com/health/pharmacology/
library/weekly/aa970710.htm

Source: 1
Navigation: 1
Interactivity: 1
Overall: 1

About.com has an enormous amount of medical information, most of it extremely useful and well written. This particular page deals with Parkinson's disease drugs. Here you will find most likely the longest list of Parkinson's drugs and explanations anywhere on the Web. You can read about new drug approvals, as well as post or read messages on the message board. Also, take advantage of the many links within the page and learn about drug interactions. If you have questions about why doctors prescribe certain medications, this is your site.

American Parkinson Disease Association
www.apdaparkinson.com

Source: 1
Navigation: 2
Interactivity: 1
Overall: 1

This site provides basic Parkinson's information without burdening its visitors with overly scientific information. You can order, or download for free, several booklets that deal with Parkinson's. By clicking on the support link, you'll be taken to a map of the United States that then allows you to click on your state and find the nearest support groups. The site also offers a host of links that connect you to some of the best sites on the Web. This simple site won't overwhelm you, but it can provide some valuable assistance.

Michael J. Fox Foundation
www.michaeljfox.org

Source: 2
Navigation: 3
Interactivity: 1
Overall: 2

This site shows what a famous name and big money can do in service of others: create an extremely user-friendly, well-advised information depot. Michael J. Fox has drawn great content contributors who provide excellent information that's written for everyone to understand. This site is all about the consumer and getting the word out.

National Institute of Neurological Disorders and Stroke
www.ninds.nih.gov/health_and_medical/disorder_
    index.htm

Source: 3
Navigation: 3
Interactivity: 1
Overall: 2

This site belongs to one of the institutes run by the government's National Institutes of Health, and, like its other sites, has the same high quality of information. The site is designed with the public in mind, so it keeps the content at a level that can be easily understood without compromising the scientific credibility. There isn't much in the way of interactivity, but the links will lead you to the best sites on the Net. This site is sure to fulfill your information needs in a hurry.

National Parkinson Foundation
www.parkinson.org

Source: 3
Navigation: 2
Interactivity: 2
Overall: 3

This is the website of one of the best Parkinson's organizations in the world. The information, as you would expect, is plentiful and well presented. The fact sheets address all types of issues from surgical treatment to nutritional guidelines. You can ask the medical director of the foundation a question, or you can check out the public forum and discuss Parkinsonian issues with patients and health professionals.

Parkinson's Disease Foundation
www.pdf.org

Source: 2
Navigation: 2
Interactivity: 1
Overall: 2

This is a site that will take you from A to Z on Parkinson's, and it does it in such a way that learning is effortless. The site is well organized and directs you to exactly where you need to be to gather specific information. You can also pop a question to the expert and read other people's questions and answers. The links are some of the best on the Net. This is a great starting point to learn about Parkinson's.

Parkinson's Institute
www.parkinsonsinstitute.org

Source: 3
Navigation: 2
Interactivity: 1
Overall: 1

This site is heavily dedicated to research on Parkinson's disease, but it also contains enough basic information about the disease to make it worth your while to stop by. The information that is consumer-friendly isn't as extensive as that offered by some of the other sites, but you will leave with a basic understanding of the disease. One advantage of this site is that it also deals with other movement disorders, so while you're here you can learn about related diseases.

Parkinson Society Canada
www.parkinson.ca

Source: 1
Navigation: 3
Interactivity: 2
Overall: 1

This Canadian site is written in English, and its tidy organization makes it extremely easy to navigate. You will be given a crash course on Parkinson's and the potential treatments. You can also read the stories of other sufferers and share your own.

The message board is quite active, with postings covering a range of topics. It's easy to spend a lot of time at this site.

We Move: Worldwide Education and Awareness for
    Movement Disorders
www.wemove.org

Source: 2
Navigation: 2
Interactivity: 3
Overall: 2

This site deals with several of the movement disorders, including Parkinson's. It has an enormous amount of information to offer consumers beyond the basics. You can participate in a chat room or read the transcripts from previous chats. If that's not enough, check out some of the webcast presentations. The site will also link you to the sites of several leading organizations and advocacy groups.

World Parkinson Disease Association
www.wpda.org

Source: 1
Navigation: 2
Interactivity: 1
Overall: 1

This site will give you an overview of Parkinson's without weighing you down with overly scientific information. The home page runs a breathtaking list of articles that cover all types of Parkinson's-related issues, especially treatment. If you want to know what's going on in the world of research, the site has some of that also. This site is best used when you want to read the latest Parkinson's headlines.

Plastic Surgery

American Society for Aesthetic Plastic Surgery
www.surgery.org

Source: 2
Navigation: 3
Interactivity: 1
Overall: 2

If you are interested in cosmetic surgery, this is a good site on which to find general information, FAQs, and even surgery indications for men! The site provides some helpful descriptions of surgeries with pictures. Some might find the glamour shots on the home page a drawback.

Medem
www.medem.com

Source: 3
Navigation: 3
Interactivity: 1
Overall: 3

This is a valuable resource for patients seeking information about reconstructive or cosmetic procedures. The site is sponsored by the medical societies of board-certified specialists and contains peer-reviewed information. If you are looking for general to advanced information about any medical topic, this is a great place to start your search.

Plastic Surgery Information Service
www.plasticsurgery.org

Source: 3
Navigation: 3

Interactivity: 1
Overall: 3

This is probably the best site for information on specific plastic surgery procedures, statistics, and physician referral. The site is sponsored by the American Society of Plastic Surgeons and the Plastic Surgery Educational Fund and therefore makes every effort to post only the most reliable information.

Podiatry

California Podiatric Medical Association
www.podiatrists.org/bluebook_index.htm

Source: 3
Navigation: 2
Interactivity: 1
Overall: 2

This is a good site on podiatry with some very helpful links. The site is really simple and broken down so that anyone can understand what a podiatrist does and why he or she is so important. It's a bit self-promotional, but the main focus is still on the consumer looking for answers. You'll leave the site with a clearer understanding of the importance of taking care of your feet.

Dr Foot
www.drfoot.co.uk

Source: 3
Navigation: 1

Interactivity: 2
Overall: 2

This U.K. website is very helpful. It's an informative site that is easily broken down by foot subject. It's updated frequently and is user-friendly. But be prepared to scroll! For anyone looking for information on warts, be advised that the term "verrucae" is commonly used in the United Kingdom.

Feet for Life
www.feetforlife.org

Source: 3
Navigation: 2
Interactivity: 1
Overall: 3

This is a really informative site for general foot questions. And although it's a U.K. website, the information found on feet is just as valuable here as across the pond. You do, however, have to navigate the site a bit to find what you're looking for.

Foot & Ankle Link Library
www.footandankle.com/podmed

Source: N/A
Navigation: N/A
Interactivity: N/A
Overall: 2

This site is a bit different from others reviewed because it's simply a site of links. I list it here because its links to podiatric organizations, education on podiatry, and where to find products for the feet, among other things, can be quickly accessed with the click of a mouse. Using this site may require some patience, as some of the links do not seem to function properly. Still, it's worth a gander.

PodiatryChannel
www.podiatrychannel.com

Source: 3
Navigation: 3
Interactivity: 3
Overall: 3

If you're looking for the mother of all podiatry websites, this is it. It's both helpful and simple. With its small font, it's easy to think the site is overwhelming because of the content. Not so. You can connect to information on nearly every type of foot ailment with a single click from the home page. Everything from finding a podiatrist to joining an online chat is right here, including occasional live chat forums with selected discussion topics.

PodiatryNetwork.com
www.podiatrynetwork.com

Source: 3
Navigation: 3
Interactivity: 1
Overall: 3

This site is a breath of fresh air, providing very useful articles in addition to all you need to know about basic foot disorders and how to go about rectifying them. It's simple and unpretentious. And that's how the site's creators want it to be. Information on how to find the right doctor is found on the same page as how to pick the right shoe. Both doctors and laypeople are encouraged to take advantage of this site.

Podiatry Online
www.footdoc.com

Source: 3
Navigation: 1
Interactivity: 1
Overall: 2

Why would I recommend a site that's only for members? I do
so because the information available to the general public is
very useful. By using the archive located at the bottom right-
hand corner of the page, you're sure to find a link to an article
or some general information about what you're looking for.
The site is a forum for podiatrists, but the novice can still find
pertinent information with regard to the foot.

Reproductive Health
(Also see **Obstetrics and Gynecology.**)

American College of Obstetricians and Gynecologists
www.acog.org

Source: 3
Navigation: 3
Interactivity: 1
Overall: 3

This is a good site from which to gather peer-reviewed information on more than 150 reproductive health topics. Information is organized from introductory to advanced/professional
research. Some of the advanced or professional articles may be
difficult reading.

Family Health International
www.fhi.org

Source: 2
Navigation: 3
Interactivity: 1
Overall: 2

The Family Health International site provides a range of information on reproductive health in several languages and contains helpful information for parents wanting to discuss sex with their children. It's not the only stop you should make on the Net, but it could prove to be an informative one.

The Journal of the American Medical Association
    Women's Health Information Center
www.ama-assn.org/special/womh/womh.htm

Source: 3
Navigation: 3
Interactivity: 1
Overall: 2

This is an authoritative site on women's health issues, backed by one of the most credible medical associations and journals in the world. Some information may be difficult to understand by the lay reader; however, if you take the time to search, you'll be delighted by what you'll find.

MayoClinic.com
www.mayoclinic.com/home?id=4.1.6

Source: 3
Navigation: 3
Interactivity: 1
Overall: 3

This is a good site on which to start your search on reproductive health. It is well organized and easy to navigate. The information is also easy to read and understand. The site is regularly reviewed and updated by Mayo Clinic researchers and physicians, making this site an authoritative source.

National Women's Health Resource Center
www.healthywomen.org

Source: 3
Navigation: 3
Interactivity: 1
Overall: 3

This site is well organized and easy to navigate. Each topic contains references, and all content is reviewed by medical professionals. The site uses only peer-reviewed, reputable journals, as well as books published recently by experts. It is concise and easy to understand.

Planned Parenthood
www.plannedparenthood.org

Source: 3
Navigation: 2
Interactivity: 1
Overall: 3

This site contains comprehensive information on a variety of reproductive topics, including how to talk to your kids about sex, menopause, sexuality, pregnancy, and sexually transmitted diseases.

ReproLine: Reproductive Health Online
www.reproline.jhu.edu

Source: 3
Navigation: 3
Interactivity: 1
Overall: 3

This very helpful site is an affiliate of Johns Hopkins University and is designed for people needing in-depth information about reproductive health. It includes multimedia material and is presented in a well-organized, easy-to-read format.

Siecus
www.siecus.org

Source: 2
Navigation: 3
Interactivity: 1
Overall: 2

This easy-to-understand, well-organized site is a great resource for parents. It's the electronic face of a nonprofit organization dedicated to developing, collecting, and disseminating information about sexual health. It covers topics such as sexual education, HIV/AIDS, and adolescent abstinence. You'll also find fact sheets that deal with different types of sexuality questions such as gay and lesbian relationships and teenage pregnancy.

Women's Health Interactive
www.womens-health.com

Source: 2
Navigation: 3

> *Interactivity: 1*
> *Overall: 3*

This site is thorough and easy to navigate. It contains comprehensive, clear information. It also has really good graphics and a pleasing design. You'll read information on everything from effective birth control to an entire group of pages dedicated to a fertility center and a separate reproductive center. This site is tailor-made for research into women's health and reproductive issues. You'll find lots of important information.

Respiratory Diseases/Emphysema/Chronic Obstructive Pulmonary Disease

> American Lung Association
> www.lungusa.org
>
> *Source: 3*
> *Navigation: 3*
> *Interactivity: 2*
> *Overall: 3*

Don't look any further than this site for high-quality, trustworthy information. It has easy-to-use, thorough data in all categories of respiratory problems, as well as current news. It's great to scroll through the disease categories, which are so specific they'll almost certainly educate you and make you feel as if the site is geared toward you personally.

> Australian Lung Foundation
> www.lungnet.org.au
>
> *Source: 3*
> *Navigation: 2*

Interactivity: 2
Overall: 2

This is an excellent learning site, and one that is particularly easy to use. I especially enjoyed the description of how the lungs work, which is thorough and well written. It is a great place to start and then scroll down to more specific subsections on various lung problems. They deal with simple, yet important questions and answer them very well. Particularly strong is an easy-to-access section on COPD.

British Thoracic Society
www.brit-thoracic.org.uk

Source: 3
Navigation: 2
Interactivity: 1
Overall: 2

This is a nicely sectioned site on respiratory diseases, and it contains detailed information on various lung diseases. One problem, however, is that the information is simply not as easy to read as on other sites. Still, this is a very credible site and the information can be quite helpful once you find what you're looking for.

Chronic Lung Disease Forum
www.cheshire-med.com/programs/pulrehab/forum/
    cldform.html

Source: 1
Navigation: 3
Interactivity: 3
Overall: 2

If you're looking for interactive learning and want to read other people's stories, this is a great site to visit. Totally free of ads, this site is simply a forum with quality messages and a search function so you can find what you are looking for. It is thorough, the site is updated many times a day, and searches are easy. In addition there is a chat function and suggested chat times to help initiate meetings.

Emphysema Foundation for Our Right to Survive
www.emphysema.net

Source: 2
Navigation: 3
Interactivity: 2
Overall: 3

If you have a question or need to know something about emphysema/COPD; if you are looking for real-life stories by people coping with this disease; or if you are searching for news stories, this site has it all. It is very comprehensive, providing answers to any questions you may have while keeping you involved through free newsletters and e-mails about events. It might prove to be the beginning, middle, and end of your search about this condition.

Living with COPD
www.papapoo.com

Source: 1
Navigation: 2
Interactivity: 2
Overall: 2

Do *not* make this the first site you visit to learn about COPD. *Do* visit this site for support. You can read other people's stories, essays by patients, and advice from people who have the disease. With its COPD humor section, this site succeeds in showing that a little laughter hurts no one.

The National Emphysema Foundation
www.emphysemafoundation.org

Source: 3
Navigation: 3
Interactivity: 2
Overall: 2

This is an excellent preventive and educational site on which to start your research, with interactive learning and suggestions for great ways to care for your lungs before anything happens. And as it goes on to discuss COPD and asthma, it is extremely detailed, telling and showing you what to expect regarding symptoms, tests, and treatments.

No Air to Go
http://noairtogo.tripod.com

Source: 2
Navigation: 2
Interactivity: 3
Overall: 2

This is a highly interactive site with no shortage of information. You'll find extensive definitions of terms as well as credible links that are only a click away. The site's strengths are an active forum, chat rooms, and an abundance of articles directed toward the patient population. This site is dedicated to your use, and the only problem can be the sometimes annoying pop-up ads for tripod.com.

Senior Health

About.com on Senior Health
www.seniorhealth.about.com/mbody.htm

Source: 3
Navigation: 3
Interactivity: 3
Overall: 3

This is one of the best sites on the Net covering senior health concerns. As are most of About.com's sites, it's absolutely full of excellent articles that cover almost any topic you can think of. It is organized efficiently, and the interactive component is tremendously useful and easy to join. You can participate in live chats with other seniors or health professionals or read postings from a discussion forum. Simply put, you won't get much better than this when looking for senior health information on the Net.

AgeNet Eldercare Network
www.agenet.com

Source: 2
Navigation: 3
Interactivity: 1
Overall: 2

If you want to read breaking senior health news or a reviews on a specific medical condition, you'll be pleased with what this site has to offer. It's written with the consumer in mind, and the information is accessible and well organized. You can ask an expert a question or plug into the caregiver tools and read an eldercare checklist. This site gives you great information on senior health and beyond.

American Association of Retired Persons
www.aarp.org/healthguide

Source: 2
Navigation: 3
Interactivity: 3
Overall: 3

The AARP is the country's largest organization for retired people. It's well known for its financial and political clout, and it ought to be known also for the health content on its website. The full list of health and wellness issues that aging people face is addressed in a well-organized and easy-to-follow manner. Join the discussion center and learn about ways to remain calm. Plug into the fitness center and learn how to keep in shape. Simply put, this site is loaded, and it has something for everyone.

American Geriatrics Society
www.americangeriatrics.org

Source: 3
Navigation: 3
Interactivity: 1
Overall: 2

This is the home of one of the most respected organizations that deals with aging-related issues. Some of the site is accessible only to members (for a fee), but the consumer health information is free. By clicking the education link, you'll find an extremely long list of articles on a variety of topics from osteo-porosis to depression. These articles are written by medical professionals for consumers. They are easy to read and full of valuable information. You can also use the excellent links it has to other websites to continue your search for information.

CBS HealthWatch Senior Health Center
www.cbshealthwatch.medscape.com/seniorhealthcenter

Source: 2
Navigation: 3
Interactivity: 2
Overall: 2

This site is refreshing and full of important senior health infor-mation that sheds light on a variety of senior-related issues. The content is provided by Medscape, a respected and trusted source of medical information. You can read the basics or choose the news headlines that cover several senior health is-sues. There's also an opportunity to chat live with a nurse or ask about available senior services. Those of you who speak Span-ish, don't feel left out, because the site has a host of pages for you also.

ElderWeb: Body & Soul
www.elderweb.com/body&soul

Source: 2
Navigation: 3
Interactivity: 1
Overall: 2

While this site addresses many senior issues, it also allots a great deal of space to health. It's full of important health information covering a wide range of topics. Instead of fact sheets, you're offered the latest headlines and articles covering the health topic of your choice. Most of these articles draw from peer-reviewed medical journals and present the information in a way that's easy to follow. You'll be surprised at how complicated topics can be made easy to understand.

MEDLINEplus on Seniors' Health
www.nlm.nih.gov/medlineplus/
   seniorshealthgeneral.html

Source: 3
Navigation: 3
Interactivity: 1
Overall: 3

If you're looking for the best information on senior health topics, you can't go wrong with these pages from the National Library of Medicine. The site is well organized and chock full of information covering more conditions than you could probably dream up. The power of this site is the extensive and first-rate quality resources that back it. There's a good chance that once you come here, you won't need to type in another URL for the rest of your search.

National Aging Information Center
www.aoa.gov/naic

Source: 1
Navigation: 2
Interactivity: 2
Overall: 1

This site isn't strictly devoted to geriatric health issues, as it also contains information about several other aging issues. The health information it does contain, however, is well written and credible. Most of the content comes from other sources, written by experts in each disease. A little work is required to search for the information, but the effort is well worth it.

National Institute on Aging
www.nih.gov/nia

Source: 3
Navigation: 2
Interactivity: 1
Overall: 2

This site is full of excellent, well-written information; the problem is finding it. Unfortunately, the site doesn't list all of the diseases and conditions it covers. Instead, you must use the publications link and search for the information desired. This isn't the most convenient or effective way to do research, but once you find what you're looking for, you'll find that the information is of excellent quality.

New York State Office for the Aging
www.agingwell.state.ny.us

Source: 3
Navigation: 3
Interactivity: 1
Overall: 3

This is a wonderful site for senior health. It is one of the best-designed sites I've seen and is very appealing visually. The home page is divided into several sections ranging from health and safety to eating well. The information is easy to read and amazingly comprehensive. This site has enough information that you can virtually lose yourself in it and enjoy every minute. It makes looking for information fun and extremely convenient.

Sexual Health

Go Ask Alice on Sexual Health
www.goaskalice.columbia.edu/Cat7.html

Source: 3
Navigation: 2
Interactivity: 1
Overall: 2

This is not the prettiest site or the easiest to navigate, as all the information is initially on one page, yet the breadth of information is enormous, with a great many questions answered thoroughly and expertly by Columbia physicians and educators. The information is reader-friendly and in a "Dear Alice" format to arouse more interest.

Glass Wings: Sensual Celebrations
www.glasswings.com/au/sexual/celebrations.html

Source: 1
Navigation: 2
Interactivity: 2
Overall: 2

If you're looking not for factual information but for help with getting more in touch with your sexuality, being comfortable with your body, and becoming at ease talking about sex, this is a great site. It offers interesting articles and stories with topics such as feminism and rape, humorous stories, and even the famous "Miller's Tale" from Chaucer's *Canterbury Tales.*

SexualHealth.com
www.sexualhealth.com

Source: 2
Navigation: 3
Interactivity: 2
Overall: 2

This is a great educational site with something for everyone. The range of subsections is extremely vast, and the information provided is expert. The great thing about this site is that most of the information is provided through answers to specific questions, and the broad range of topics means that there are a great number of questions and answers.

ThriveOnline on Sexuality
http://thriveonline.oxygen.com/sex/index.html

Source: 2
Navigation: 3
Interactivity: 3
Overall: 2

This is an easy-to-use site that is updated on a daily basis. Not only is it good for all sorts of answers on sexual health questions, but it also offers chats about such topics as the art of flirting. The forums are lively and interesting too. The categories are interactive, making it a fun, yet informative site. It makes one feel that discussing sexual health is easy and should be comfortable.

www.iwannaknow.org
www.iwannaknow.org

Source: 3
Navigation: 3
Interactivity: 3
Overall: 2

Come here if you're a teen looking for a credible site to educate yourself on sexual health. It's particularly great for teens because of its great "Quick Facts" section, through which the ever-impatient teen can get the question he or she needs answered fast. Beyond that, the information is decent and a chat room is available for use at designated after-school times.

Skin Disorders
See **Dermatology/Skin Disorders.**

Sleep Disorders

About.com on Sleep Disorders
www.sleepdisorders.about.com

Source: 2
Navigation: 3
Interactivity: 3
Overall: 2

The site is separated into categories within which well-organized information is available. It is updated frequently by way of "spotlights," which highlight new developments, and contains a forum and chat room, through which a great number of issues are discussed frequently. It is a very public-friendly site. Most of the articles back up arguments with studies and quotes.

American Academy of Sleep Medicine
www.asda.org

Source: 3
Navigation: 2
Interactivity: 1
Overall: 2

Though the site has valuable information, going through the irrelevant items to find out where you need to go may be frustrating at first. However, once you're in, the categories are well described and the general introduction, especially to troubles with sleep, is especially well written and very informative. The links here are high quality, and the site is set up by a well-qualified staff.

MEDLINEplus on Sleep Disorders
www.nlm.nih.gov/medlineplus/sleepdisorders.html

Source: 3
Navigation: 2
Interactivity: 1
Overall: 2

This compilation site, composed of many great links, makes the search for sleep information easier on you, the patient, by providing you credible, easy-to-find information. Though the site may seem slightly intimidating at first, it is comforting to know that it has done some of the Web browsing for you and may be able to direct you on the right path to the information you are seeking.

National Institutes of Health National Center on Sleep
    Disorders Research
www.nhlbi.nih.gov/about/ncsdr/

Source: 3
Navigation: 1

Interactivity: 1
Overall: 1

The NIH remains one of the most highly regarded institutions in the medical world, yet this site is lacking in depth and breadth of information and the PDF format, which requires Adobe Acrobat Reader to read, may make the articles more difficult for some to access. Apart from one interactive quiz, interactivity is definitely lacking.

National Sleep Foundation
www.sleepfoundation.org

Source: 3
Navigation: 2
Interactivity: 2
Overall: 2

This is a frequently updated, very credible site, with categories involving the various sleep disorders and articles that are well written, easy to read, and extremely informative. The operators of the site are professionals and provide you access to further information within each different sleep disorder you search. A free newsletter keeps you updated.

SleepDisorders.com
www.sleepdisorders.com

Source: 2
Navigation: 1
Interactivity: 1
Overall: 1

This site, updated monthly, is organized into categories of sleep disorders, and many quality links to other sites give you direct access to their articles. If you are searching for one site to guide you in your search and educate you in specific areas, this is a good site. Ads pop up occasionally, a definite annoyance, and something that must be dealt with if you access this site.

Sleepnet.com
www.sleepnet.com

Source: 2
Navigation: 3
Interactivity: 3
Overall: 2

This well-organized site categorizes the various sleep disorders for easier research, yet the information is not the strongest part of this site. The forums are the only part of the site that are up-dated frequently, and they are of the most use. The posts are both thoughtful and insightful, as patients display much care in and attention to what they write.

Sports Medicine/Fitness

About.com on Sports Medicine
www.orthopedics.about.com/cs/sportsmedicine

Source: 2
Navigation: 2
Interactivity: 1
Overall: 2

This site is very well organized into categories of sports medicine relating to different body parts as well as different surgeries; it contains info ranging from the very general to the very specific. It is definitely a good place to begin your research, and it would be a good place to end it if only it contained more updates and news so that you could keep coming back. Nonetheless, for background research this is a good place to go; it will give you the fundamentals you need.

American Sports Medicine Institute
www.asmi.org

Source: 3
Navigation: 1
Interactivity: 3
Overall: 2

This is not the easiest site to work through due to the fact that most of the resources are accessed through links to medical and scientific journals; however, if you are looking for a site to begin an advanced search about sports medicine issues, this is an important one. It will make your job easier by simply directing you to different journals and allowing you to choose. But remember this is best only if you want to begin an advanced search.

CBS HealthWatch Sports Medicine and Fitness Center
www.cbshealthwatch.medscape.com/
      sportsmedicinecenter

Source: 3
Navigation: 3
Interactivity: 2
Overall: 3

This is an extremely easy to use site and can be a guide you not only start with but continue to visit. It covers the basics well, in a simple yet thorough format that gives you a strong foundation, and builds on it daily with new tips and answers to questions many people like yourself have had. The site is very complete and it demonstrates a real understanding of what you need. You can also ask experts questions and participate in discussions.

Fitness Center
www.justmove.org/home.cfm

Source: 3
Navigation: 3
Interactivity: 3
Overall: 3

Run by the American Heart Association, this site will keep you informed, teach you the basics, and allow you to actively maintain and monitor your own health and progress. It is a fun place to be and an informative one as well—overall an encouraging site. In addition, its discussion forums include many topics and are very thoughtful. Visit the site as you begin planning your workouts, then continue to visit it afterward to stay up to date with health news.

The Physician and Sportsmedicine Online
www.physsportsmed.com/personal.htm

Source: 3
Navigation: 2
Interactivity: 1
Overall: 3

This online health journal is the apex of sports medicine information with a wide variety of detailed, credible articles arranged in categories ranging from lifestyle to rehabilitation to equipment and apparel. It is an excellent place if you really wish to become a more aware person in terms of fitness, prevention, and even consumerism.

Shape Up America!
www.shapeup.org

Source: 3
Navigation: 2
Interactivity: 3
Overall: 3

This is an excellent site for those looking for fitness and nutrition advice and information. The information, I feel, is not as strong as that on some other sites, yet it is sufficient. The site's strength, however, is its interactivity. In particular, the cyber-kitchen is extremely enjoyable as well as useful, as it takes your personal characteristics and desires and molds a diet plan for you personally. The discussion areas are also strong and will definitely provide you with good ideas.

Stroke

American Stroke Association
www.strokeassociation.org
American Heart Association: Heart and Stroke A–Z
    Guide: www.americanheart.org

Source: 3
Navigation: 3
Interactivity: 1
Overall: 3

Visit this site for an extensive A-to-Z glossary listing of heart and stroke terms as well as a 2001 Statistical Update and 2001 Biostatistical Fact Sheet. Each term links you to a simple description. The index is good if you know what you're looking for—not so good if you are just looking to browse and learn.

BBC Online Health: The Stroke Guide
www.bbc.co.uk/health/stroke/about.shtml

Source: 3
Navigation: 2
Interactivity: 2
Overall: 2

This is an outstanding layperson's introduction to stroke from the British Broadcasting Corporation. It's a portion of a much larger health site, so don't be distracted by the other conditions listed on the top and left-hand navigation bars—just focus on the stroke information on the middle and right-hand side of this page. The navigation bar items are in a small font, but it will be worth your while to click on the different areas of the stroke guide.

Heart Information Network
www.heartinfo.org

Source: 2
Navigation: 2
Interactivity: 2
Overall: 2

This is a site for overall heart health, of which high blood pressure, cholesterol, and stroke are ingredients. There are a lot of search options, and if you know what you're looking for, the odds are that you'll get some answers on this site. It's a bit confusing to navigate, and the stroke information won't hit you in the face . . . but after doing a bit of searching, I think you'll find some valuable information. The nutrition guide, question-and-answer library, and many search functions make the site very useful. The "Ask Us" section enables members to ask questions of physician medical advisers.

Internet Stroke Center at Washington University
www.strokecenter.org

Source: 3
Navigation: 2
Interactivity: 1
Overall: 2

This site, which provides stroke information for patients and families, is full of valuable material. Everything is clearly presented, and you'll find valuable information about stroke, feature sections on living with stroke, medications, and caregivers, and a lot of resources and links in the "directory." Recent news about stroke research is also provided.

Mayo Clinic: Division of Cerebrovascular Diseases
www.mayo.edu/cerebro/education/stroke.html

Source: 3
Navigation: 3
Interactivity: 1
Overall: 2

This is a very clear, well-organized presentation about stroke's causes, effects, diagnosis, and treatment. The patient educational content is fabulous, as is the impressive list of resources (publications) offered. This is an excellent site to learn about stroke; I'd recommend you check it out.

MedicineNet.com on Stroke
www.focusonhighbloodpressure.com/script/main/
    art.asp?articlekey=489

Source: 2
Navigation: 2

Interactivity: 1
Overall: 2

This site provides an excellent discussion on the ABCs of stroke in the main article, "Stroke." The real gems are in the right-hand navigation bar, where you can read about Stroke Related Diseases and Conditions, Stroke Related Procedures & Tests, Stroke Related Medications, Stroke Related Health Facts, Stroke Related Doctors' Views & Updates, and The Doctors' Responses. These areas are more specific and interesting, while the main article provides the basics.

National Institute of Neurological Disorders and Stroke
www.ninds.nih.gov/health_and_medical/disorders/
    stroke.htm

Source: 3
Navigation: 3
Interactivity: 1
Overall: 2

This is really a stroke fact sheet rather than an entire website by the NINDS of the National Institutes of Health; however, I decided to include it as it is highly credible and very easy to read, and provides other valuable resources. You'll find quick, trustworthy facts about the illness and its prognosis and treatment from the National Institutes of Health. The NIH is always a good resource for health topics. Credible references, organizations, and publications are listed clearly (and directly linked to) at the bottom of the fact sheet. Get the basics here before you move out into the Net.

National Stroke Association
www.stroke.org

Source: 3
Navigation: 3
Interactivity: 1
Overall: 2

The National Stroke Association does a fabulous job with its website, offering information on prevention, treatment, and caregiving. The section "All About Stroke" is very comprehensive and impressive, as is, in fact, the entire site. I wish they would stop soliciting for their newsletter and magazine, though!

StrokeHelp.com
www.strokehelp.com

Source: 3
Navigation: 3
Interactivity: 1
Overall: 1

The name of this website is very fitting—it *is* helpful for those seeking further resources on stroke or caring for those following a stroke. However, unless I missed it, there is actually no information about stroke itself. This is a good place to stop to buy educational videos on stroke and caregiving or learn about educational workshops being offered, but don't stop here if you want instant information on the condition. There are good links out, but you probably won't stay on the site for too long. The information is available in six languages.

Teen Health, General

Academy for Adolescent Health
www.healthyteens.com

Source: 2
Navigation: 2
Interactivity: 2
Overall: 2

This is a youth-friendly website that through its "Youth Connections" section provides solutions to various problems teens may face in their lives. The advice is clearly and succinctly presented to teens, with phone numbers included in case more information is desired. The only downside to the site is that the appearance seems almost childish and is not necessarily something a teen might relate to.

Adolescence Directory On-Line
http://education.indiana.edu/cas/adol/adol.html

Source: 3
Navigation: 2
Interactivity: 1
Overall: 2

This is an excellent site that is easy to search and has organized its information into categories ranging from acne to obesity to sexual abuse. Contains useful links and articles that guide you easily through the issues you wish to learn more about.

Adolescent Health Center
www.adhc.org

Source: 2
Navigation: 2

Interactivity: 1
Overall: 2

The site provides information about different issues facing teens in a simple way, to help them understand their situation better and perhaps not feel so alone. I particularly liked the segment on pregnancy, which tells an expectant mother exactly what will be occurring in her body over the three trimesters of pregnancy.

American Medical Association: Adolescent Health
   Online
www.ama-assn.org/ama/pub/category/1947.html

Source: 3
Navigation: 1
Interactivity: 1
Overall: 2

Brought to you by the nation's authority on health care, this site provides information and stats on various health issues concerning adolescents. The site is not, however, really conducive to adolescent use, due to the numerous statistically based articles and the lack of in-depth, thoughtful articles. In addition, its range of topics is limited; only a select few are covered by the site. Nonetheless, this is a wonderful resource for adults who want medical information about teens.

Centers for Disease Control and Prevention
   on Adolescent and School Health
www.cdc.gov/nccdphp/dash/

Source: 3
Navigation: 1
Interactivity: 1
Overall: 2

This is a site dedicated to both education about adolescent health and policy in educational curriculums. Yet it is not a site one should go to except to catch a glimpse of the problems and symptoms within the adolescent community. The articles are general and not extremely thoughtful, and it does not seem as though any of them would catch an adolescent's interest.

World College Health
www.worldcollegehealth.org

Source: 3
Navigation: 3
Interactivity: 1
Overall: 3

This is a site dedicated to a wide range of adolescent health issues such as learning disabilities and coping with grief. The columns are written by experts in their fields in ways directed especially toward teens to really affect their thoughts. Much more than simple stats are presented; stories are told. The only downside is the lack of updates, as new articles take a long time to appear on the site.

Transplants

American Association of Tissue Banks
www.aatb.org

Source: 1
Navigation: 2
Interactivity: 1
Overall: 1

This website won't have you raving, but it will give you some important transplant information. The FAQs are good on the basic information about transplantation, and if they don't satisfy your hunger, try the links. They're a great way to build on the knowledge you've already acquired at this site.

Children's Organ Transplant Association
www.cota.org

Source: 1
Navigation: 3
Interactivity: 1
Overall: 2

This site may be of significant assistance to parents of children in need of transplants. It offers assistance and services for people in need and provides an excellent list of links to transplant information from other sources. If you want to become a donor, this site can also tell you how to give. There isn't hard scientific information here, but its help might save a life.

LifeNet
www.tissue.org

Source: 3
Navigation: 3
Interactivity: 1
Overall: 2

This tissue bank is responsible for procuring and delivering donated tissues to hospitals and ultimately to patients. The website clearly explains what its role is in tissue donation and how one goes about getting involved from either the donor or recipient end. The stories of others who have gone through the process are informative and inspirational. The site's links are a great way to visit other organizations involved in transplantation.

National Marrow Donor Program
www.marrow.org

Source: 2
Navigation: 3
Interactivity: 1
Overall: 2

This site is excellent for those in need of or wanting to donate bone marrow. In a well-organized, easy-to-follow style, it lays out for visitors the process of donating as well as the process of receiving. The FAQs are excellent, and each major topic has its own FAQs section. You can also stop by the media room (even if you're not a journalist) and read the latest headlines. If a bone marrow transplant is in your future, this website should be high on your list of information sources.

National Transplant Assistance Fund
www.transplantfund.org

Source: 2
Navigation: 3
Interactivity: 1
Overall: 2

This site deals with one of the most important issues surrounding transplantation—how you will pay for it. You can find tips from fund-raising to deciding if moving closer to a transplant center is in your best interest. The site is well organized and constantly gives you an opportunity to contact the organization for assistance. The links are good, especially those that go to other patients' websites that discuss personal stories dealing with transplantation. Stop here—the benefits and information are about more than just the money.

National Transplant Society
www.organdonor.org

Source: 1
Navigation: 2
Interactivity: 2
Overall: 1

This site has potential, but most of it deals with encouraging donations and little with telling people how they can actually receive an organ. Organ donation is important, of course, which explains why the site heavily solicits you to become a donor. To that end, the site serves its purpose. However, its scope is quite limited, which means that you'll have to visit another site for more in-depth info. Before leaving, try the LifeChat and talk with others who may be sharing your concerns or experiences.

New England Organ Bank
www.neob.org

Source: 2
Navigation: 2
Interactivity: 1
Overall: 2

This might be a regional site, but its information is global. You are given not only statistics about different transplants but fact sheets on the major ones. You will gain a better understanding of the complicated transplantation process. As on most of the transplant sites, you can read stories of people who donated as well as those on a waiting list. Not including this site on your research journey could be a mistake.

U.S. Department of Health and Human Services: Organ
    Donation
www.organdonor.gov

Source: 3
Navigation: 3
Interactivity: 1
Overall: 2

This is a full transplantation site that addresses most issues related to transplantation. It has an interesting statistics page that gives you the number of patients waiting for different organs. It also has information on how you can become a donor. The links to other important transplantation sites and organizations are excellent. This is an important site.

TransWeb.org
transweb.org

Source: 2
Navigation: 3
Interactivity: 2
Overall: 2

If you want to know about the process of receiving an organ or donating, this site breaks it all down for you in plain English. If you want to read other people's stories, they're here. If you want links to other websites or resources, they're here. If you want info about transplantation, it's here. This site is a must-visit on your quest for transplantation information. Also, check out the links to support groups.

United Network for Organ Sharing
www.unos.org

Source: 3
Navigation: 3
Interactivity: 2
Overall: 3

This is the ultimate transplantation site. I can't think of what it doesn't offer. There are answers to the questions of both donors and recipients. The organ center tells you how patients are matched for organs and the steps in the process. This organization is responsible for monitoring the national waiting list around the clock. There are also great resources and Internet links. This site won't leave many questions unanswered.

Urology

American Foundation for Urologic Disease
www.afud.org

Source: 3
Navigation: 3
Interactivity: 1
Overall: 3

If you want reliable information on urologic diseases such as those that affect the kidney or bladder, you've found a gold mine. This site offers extensive coverage of conditions affecting these organs, as well as others such as the prostate and ureters. Great links send you to other informative sites that will enhance your search. Start here, and you won't be disappointed.

American Urologic Association
www.auanet.org

Source: 3
Navigation: 3
Interactivity: 1
Overall: 1

This site defines many of the urological conditions, succinctly explaining what they are in language you can understand. Throughout the site, specific conditions have links to other Net resources. Are you looking for a urologist? Check out the link for one near you. You can also share your experience with other patients through the patient support page.

Brady Urological Institute at Johns Hopkins Medical Institutions
http://prostate.urol.jhu.edu

Source: 3
Navigation: 3
Interactivity: 1
Overall: 2

Johns Hopkins Hospital is one of the best medical institutions in the world, and its urologic institute is equally impressive. Powered by the best minds and clinicians dealing with urologic diseases, this site is a special treat for patients as it gives you the best information these scientists have to offer. You will be able to understand the content, and the site is organized in a way that facilitates navigation. Here you can learn about everything from prostate cancer to an overactive bladder, as well as ongoing clinical trials in the disease of your concern.

> Cleveland Clinic Urological Institute
> www.clevelandclinic.org/urology
>
> *Source: 2*
> *Navigation: 3*
> *Interactivity: 1*
> *Overall: 2*

If you're looking for information on childhood urological problems, female infertility or incontinence, or enlarged prostate, it's all neatly bundled in this site. Part of one of the best-respected health care systems in the world, it packs a powerful punch. This is a site where you can quickly find what you need to know and trust that the information is reliable. There's also a separate section for physicians.

> Columbia-Presbyterian Medical Center Department
>   of Urology
> http://207.10.206.114
>
> *Source: 2*
> *Navigation: 3*
> *Interactivity: 1*
> *Overall: 2*

This academic site gives you the information you need to know with the smallest amount of hassle. The content is thorough and engaging, and you'll have the opportunity to chat with others sharing your condition through a support group. You can also learn about urologic diseases that affect children. Your questions will be answered in short order once you click on the appropriate link.

Digital Urology Journal
www.duj.com

Source: 3
Navigation: 3
Interactivity: 1
Overall: 3

This is a great source of patient information on a wide range of urological disorders. After entering the "Patient" section, you can click on the disease that concerns you and get yourself up to speed. The information provided will be enough for most people, but if you are looking for more, just try the links to other sites on the Net. Stopping here will be important as you collect urology-related information.

Loyola University Medical Center Department
    of Urology
www.luhs.org/depts/urology/html

Source: 3
Navigation: 3
Interactivity: 1
Overall: 2

This website contains information on a variety of urologic topics, ranging from the common prostate diseases to urinary tract infections. Loyola has a well-recognized medical center, and this site has that resource and more behind it. If you're interested in a clinical trial that might expose you to cutting-edge medications or technologies that are still being studied, click on the "clinical trials" link. This site is here to inform, and it does just that.

National Institute of Diabetes & Digestive & Kidney
    Diseases
www.niddk.nih.gov/health/urolog/urolog.htm

Source: 3
Navigation: 3
Interactivity: 1
Overall: 3

This is one of the best sites on the Web for information on urological diseases. It's constructed with you, the consumer, in
mind and it doesn't distract you with advertisements or donation requests. The content is not overly scientific, so you'll be
able to get the concepts with one read. You can read the statistics and fact sheets in Spanish if desired. It's hard to imagine
another site that provides such a complete array of urologic information.

University of Maryland Medicine on
    Urological Disorders
www.umm.edu/urology-info/about.htm

Source: 2
Navigation: 3
Interactivity: 1
Overall: 2

This is a strong site for urological information. You can read
about a vast array of diseases, and it's written for all to understand. The different disorders are conveniently listed on both
sides of the page, and you can access the information with a
simple click. The site also has a long list of links that will send
you to some of the other excellent urological sites on the Net.

UrologyChannel.com
www.urologychannel.com

Source: 3
Navigation: 3
Interactivity: 3
Overall: 3

This site is a great example of the potential of the Internet to provide quality information in a fun way. A broad spectrum of diseases is covered on this site; the content is written expertly and in a way that all can understand. The interactive tools are second to none, allowing you to chat with professionals or other people with a similar condition or concerns. Before taking advantage of the links, check out the breaking health news—you might read it here before the reporters get hold of it.

Vision

AllAboutVision.com
www.allaboutvision.com

Source: 2
Navigation: 3
Interactivity: 1
Overall: 2

This site is a cornucopia of eye information that tackles everything from computer vision syndrome to the effects of aging on the eyes. It is well organized and easy to navigate. The site has an accomplished editorial board that lends greater credence to the information. The eye anatomy chart helps you to finally understand those complicated-sounding eye terms, and the statistics page lets you know that you aren't suffering alone. This is a good place to start looking for answers.

American Academy of Ophthalmology
www.eyenet.org

Source: 3
Navigation: 2
Interactivity: 1
Overall: 2

This site belongs to one of the premier ophthalmology organizations in the world. It provides important information for both health professionals and consumers. The content is written to the level of the audience expected to be reading it. You can easily navigate your way around the site and enjoy the newsroom and its headlines or try one of the many links and take your search to other important sites.

American Optometric Association
www.aoanet.org

Source: 3
Navigation: 3
Interactivity: 1
Overall: 2

Here you'll find much important and useful information about eye diseases. There are also several well-written consumer guides that tell you everything from how to take care of your glasses to what should be expected during an eye exam. There's also a section for teachers and kids and classroom activities that stress the importance of proper eye care. This is a site the whole family can enjoy and pick up some important tips from.

American Society of Cataract and Refractive Surgery/
American Society of Ophthalmic Administrators
www.ascrs.org

Source: 2
Navigation: 3
Interactivity: 1
Overall: 2

If you want the skinny on laser eye surgery and can't seem to cut through the marketing hype, here it is. This professional association is home to the authorities on eye surgery, and its information-loaded website makes you feel empowered and knowledgeable. Having trouble finding someone to operate on your eyes? The site also offers a physician locator that can find the nearest doctor based on your zip code.

Glaucoma Foundation
www.glaucoma-foundation.org

Source: 3
Navigation: 3
Interactivity: 1
Overall: 2

This site provides the latest in-depth information on one of the most common preventable eye disorders. The site's layout makes it easy to navigate, leading consumers directly to the place where they can glean the most information. You won't be hit over the head with fancy medical terms or explanations. Instead, the simplicity and accuracy of the information only enhance the convenience of your search.

Health on the Net: Foundation Vision and EyeCare FAQ
www.hon.ch/Library/Theme/VisionFaq

Source: 1
Navigation: 3
Interactivity: 1
Overall: 1

This FAQs page belongs to one of the leading website integrity
agencies on the Internet. It has an easy-to-read, extensive list of
FAQs that cover most topics of interest to the general public.
Each topic has links to other websites for information. I was
surprised that some of these links were unavailable, considering that this is one of the guiding principles in how the organization evaluates other websites. The FAQs also haven't been
updated regularly, which stands in contradistinction to the organization's principles. These contradictions are troubling, but
the information and web links are vast and solid.

Medem Eye Health Library
www.medem.com/medlb/sub_detaillb.cfm?parent_id=
30&act=disp

Source: 3
Navigation: 3
Interactivity: 1
Overall: 3

This site is, as its name implies, an electronic library on eye information. It covers all of the common diseases that affect the
eye, presenting the information in an easy-to-read format. You
can also learn about the laser vision correction surgeries that
have become so popular over the last several years and find out
how to correct your vision with the proper contact lenses and
eyeglasses. This site contains a wealth of information that will
enrich your knowledge.

MEDLINEplus on Eyes and Vision
www.nlm.nih.gov/medlineplus/eyesandvision.html

Source: 3
Navigation: 3
Interactivity: 1
Overall: 2

Information on eye disease and related topics doesn't get more comprehensive than this. Drawing from trusted resources from around the world, this information bank provides the best from the brightest. Non–medical people are expected to be the primary consumers of the information, so the content is written for all to understand easily. This certainly should be where you begin your search on eye conditions.

National Eye Institute of the National Institutes
of Health
www.nei.nih.gov

Source: 3
Navigation: 3
Interactivity: 1
Overall: 2

You can't go wrong if you stop by this site to pick some important eye information. The site, which is designed with the consumer in mind, lays out the content links clearly and without much fanfare. You will also be linked to other websites that address eye diseases and provide important resources for those with vision problems. You can calculate your risk for vision problems, take the low-vision quiz, and scan the eye diagram before taking the "eye-q" tests. This is a comprehensive site just waiting for you to take advantage of it.

University of Michigan Kellogg Eye Center
www.kellogg.umich.edu/conditions

Source: 3
Navigation: 2
Interactivity: 1
Overall: 1

This site offers the basics on a variety of eye conditions and some of the diseases that cause them. There is an extensive list of FAQs that will likely cover at least one of the questions you have in mind. If that's not enough, check out the long list of links to online resources. You can also get some answers to those questions you've had about the latest eye surgeries. This is definitely a site to include on your cyberspace research quest.

Women's Health

The American Medical Women's Association
www.amwa-doc.org

Source: 3
Navigation: 3
Interactivity: 1
Overall: 2

This website is the Internet arm of one of the oldest and most trusted women's medical groups. As you can imagine, it provides lots of information that not only covers the basics but extends into other health-related concerns such as legal and political issues. Its "NewsFlash" bulletin is more doctor- than patient-friendly, but you can occasionally find something that appeals even to the non–medically oriented reader. A yearly membership fee gives you access to the whole site, but the site is most useful to health care professionals. Consumers will be satisfied with the free access and excellent links.

HealthWeb on Women's Health
www.healthweb.org/browse.cfm?subjectid=96

Source: 1
Navigation: 3
Interactivity: 1
Overall: 1

This is not a site to visit for basic information on different illnesses but, rather one you visit to find other sites. Its smart organization and absence of distracting ads allow you to do your business without interruption. The search engine is fast and pulls up results that include a long list of external resources. The credibility of this site is largely substantiated by the partners, a national collection of public and educational libraries. If you can't trust the National Library of Medicine and the other libraries it supports, whom can you trust?

iVillage.com on Women's Health
www.allhealth.com/library/nwh

Source: 3
Navigation: 3
Interactivity: 3
Overall: 3

There aren't many other sites that cover such an extensive spectrum of health concerns, everything from breast cancer to tai chi. The information is updated regularly and posted at the bottom of the page. The information is extremely credible and well resourced and done in partnership with the National Women's

Health Resource Center. The site is one of the most interactive, offering a variety of quizzes on different health topics that serve to challenge and educate. You can also participate in chatrooms or check out the message board. This site is the ultimate in one-stop information shopping.

> The Journal of the American Medical Association
>   Women's Health Information Center
> www.ama-assn.org/special/womh/womh.htm
>
> *Source: 3*
> *Navigation: 3*
> *Interactivity: 1*
> *Overall: 2*

This website draws on one of the most respected medical journals in the world. It gives visitors access to articles not only from *The Journal of the American Medical Association* but from other journals as well. The site is no-nonsense and doesn't distract you with excessive advertising or solicitations. I wouldn't suggest stopping here first for basic information as the site's search engine and design are more suited to the slightly more advanced Internet user. If you want to know what the latest research shows, there is no better information depot.

> MayoClinic.com Women's Center
> www.mayoclinic.com/home?id=4.1.7
>
> *Source: 3*
> *Navigation: 3*
> *Interactivity: 1*
> *Overall: 2*

The Mayo Clinic is one of the premier academic medical institutions in the world, a reputation its website upholds. The information is thoughtful and well organized, and the pages are clean. I also like how specific the site is about the diseases that it covers, which helps facilitate your search. The section showing the latest headlines is also interesting, bringing you research findings from the leading medical journals. Whether you are a man or woman, come here to learn about women's health issues.

The Merck Manual of Medical Information—Home Edition
www.merck.com/pubs/mmanual_home/contents.htm

Source: 2
Navigation: 3
Interactivity: N/A
Overall: 2

I'm not inclined to include sites that are sponsored by or owned by pharmaceutical companies, but this site has such excellent information that it's hard not to recommend it. Fortunately, there are no advertisements or drug selling. In fact, the site is really an online version of the *Merck Manual,* a well-respected source that we physicians often use. You can simply click on the chapters in section 22—Women's Health Issues—and read until your heart is content.

National Asian Women's Health Organization
www.nawho.org

Source: 1
Navigation: 2
Interactivity: 1
Overall: 1

This site's most important feature seems to be its culturally sensitive approach to Asian women's health concerns. It has a strong voice that resonates in the links and internal resources, pushing the agenda to empower, educate, and network Asian women with regard to their health. The site tends to be a little content-light, superficially glossing over subjects before linking the consumer to other sites or resources. It's not clear who provides the scientific content or how frequently it's updated, but a visit to this site can empower those who are concerned about the issues covered.

National Women's Health Information Center
www.4woman.gov

Source: 2
Navigation: 2
Interactivity: 1
Overall: 2

This site covers the wide spectrum of women's issues in a relaxed format that allows you to surf the site effortlessly. You'll find excellent information covering a range of topics from physical abuse to pregnancy. The site also offers information in Spanish and has a special link dedicated to minority health. All types of women are likely to find valuable information on this site—all you have to do is log on.

Office on Women's Health
www.4woman.gov/owh

Source: 3
Navigation: 3
Interactivity: 1
Overall: 3

This site attempts to provide information for women of all ages and colors. It draws on the vast resources of the U.S. Department of Health and Human Services and organizes the content according to specific diseases and/or a particular demographic. If you take advantage of all the available links, you can't help but leave better informed. If you want more detailed information, you can download copies of the brochures and fact sheets.

Women's Health Interactive
www.womens-health.com

Source: 2
Navigation: 3
Interactivity: 3
Overall: 2

This website delivers on its title, as it is the most interactive and user-friendly women's health website. The site is conveniently organized, which makes it easy to navigate. There is a lot of information covering a wide range of topics. The site is loaded with extras that help distinguish it from others. Use the services links to find resources for your medical condition, or enter the chat rooms for discussions with others who might share your medical illness. This well-rounded site will not only inform you but will also open the door to the vast Internet resources on women's health.

Web Resources Directory

Complementary and Alternative Medicine Sites
About.com on Alternative Medicine
www.altmedicine.about.com/mbody.htm
Alternative Medicine Channel
www.alternativemedicinechannel.com
American Cancer Society: Complementary & Alternative
Methods
www.cancer.org/alt_therapy
healthfinder
www.healthfinder.gov
National Center for Complementary and Alternative
Medicine
www.nccam.nih.gov
The Richard and Hinda Rosenthal Center for Complementary
and Alternative Medicine
http://cpmcnet.columbia.edu/dept/rosenthal
The Alternative Medicine Home Page
www.pitt.edu/~cbw/altm.html

Online Drug Information Sites
Healthtouch Online
www.healthtouch.com
MEDLINEplus: Drug Information
www.nlm.nih.gov/medlineplus/druginformation.html

PDR.net
    www.pdr.net
RxList.com
    www.rxlist.com
Safemedication.com
    www.safemedication.com

Online Medical Dictionaries
    CancerWeb
        www.graylab.ac.uk/omd
    Intellihealth: Merriam-Webster's Medical Dictionary
        www.intelihealth.com
    MedicineNet.com
        www.medterms.com/Script/Main/hp.asp
    yourDictionary.com
        www.yourdictionary.com

Acknowledgments

These names may not mean much to you, but I include them here to acknowledge their assistance, guidance, and creative energies. The order in which they appear in no way reflects any difference in my appreciation.

First, thanks to my ever-loving and supportive family, who allowed me to disappear and write this book. All of you were there for me, if not physically, then spiritually: Ma (Rena) and Noy; my amazing twin brother and excellent role model, Dana; my cousin Fred, with his words of encouragement; Triste, who actually helped me review some of these sites and gather the research without any complaints but with just love and support; my grandfather, Robert S. Cherry, a true hero, in memoriam. Also Grandma, Aunt Chris, Aunt Helen, and Aunt Dora Bee, who's unbeatable even at her advanced age; Uncle Bob, who supported me at a time in my life when no one else did; Uncle Johnny, the great educator and inspiration to succeed; Lynn, who kept me in check along the way; Aunt Bettie, who's the sweetest person I've ever met; Aunt Helen Gray, whose independence has inspired me all of my life; Billy, who continues to believe in spite of incredible odds stacked against him; Robby, who has always been in my heart despite our physical distance; Damian, who's tough on the outside but a pussycat at heart; Oosh (Richard Allen West), who I believe can do great things in life; Walkiris (Keedy), who tolerates my endless teasing and always flashes her pretty smile; little William, who continues to grow into a fine young man; Lisa, who's making a way in tough times for my little cousins; little Damian, who I hope will one day carry the torch; Dante, who as the baby of the family has brought all of us tremendous joy.

My editor supreme, Mary Bahr, has been one of the greatest driving forces behind this book. She's intelligent, indefatigable, and the greatest supporter a writer could ask for.

My friends allowed me to reschedule dinners and to not return phone calls as I raced against deadlines; their support has been unwavering: my Harvard kats, Cards (Jonathan Cardi) and Ron Mitchell; Leon Carter, successful sports editor of the New York *Daily News,* has been a confidant and true friend; Jane Freiman, my editor at the New York *Daily News,* who hired me to write my first column; Walter Isaacson, who was the editor of *Time* magazine and gave me my shot at the big time; Jim Kelly, the new and very competent editor at *Time,* who has supported me since I was hired; Philip Elmer-Dewitt, assistant managing editor of *Time* and head of the science group, whose unrivaled editing skills have made my columns appear much better after he put his deft touch to them.

Paula Walker Madison gave me my first broadcasting gig at WNBC-TV in New York City, and now she's the president and general manager of KNBC-TV in Los Angeles. Dennis Swanson, president and general manager of WNBC-TV, has taught me about the business and has supported my hectic schedule. Dianne Doctor, the current news director at the station and a collaborator, has been a big supporter. Jeff Zucker, former executive producer of NBC's *Today* show and now the president of NBC Entertainment—thanks for believing, Jeff. Susan Dutcher at *Weekend Today* never tires of me and always wants to help with my career. And thanks to Rod Prince and David Chanatry of NBC's *Weekend Nightly News*—two excellent journalists, friends, teachers, and collaborators.

Lastly, I want to thank those tireless souls who helped me check these 550 plus websites: Carl Schweitzer, whose sharp eye and intellect have made me respect him all the more; Ankur Parikh, who's now in medical school; Robert Bledsoe, who will be a star one day; Taylor Caprio, who has organized my life; my intern, Stephanie; and the ever-reliable and smart Liz Gordon. Art Norman, anchorman at NBC5 in Chicago and his wife, Ondi, gave me my first start in broadcast journalism—you both know how much you mean to me!

Index

About the Author

IAN K. SMITH, M.D., is a medical/health reporter for NBC's *Nightly News* and the *Today* show. He also writes a weekly health column for the New York *Daily News* and is a medical columnist for *Time* magazine. Dr. Smith graduated from Harvard University and earned a master's degree in science education from Columbia University. He attended Dartmouth Medical School and completed the last two years of his medical education at the University of Chicago Pritzker School of Medicine. He is also the author of *The Take-Control Diet: A Life Plan for Thinking People.* Dr. Smith currently resides in Manhattan.

About AtRandom.com Books

AtRandom.com Books is dedicated to publishing original books that harness the power of new technologies. Each title, commissioned expressly for this publishing format, will be offered simultaneously as a trade paperback and in various digital formats.

AtRandom.com books are designed to provide people with choices about their reading experience and the information they can obtain. They are aimed at defined communities of highly motivated readers who want immediate access to substantive and artful writing on the various subjects that fascinate them.

Our list features expert information on health, business, technology, politics, culture, entertainment, law, finance, travel, and a variety of other topics. Whether written in a spirit of play, rigorous critique, or practical advice, these books possess a vitality that new ways of publishing can aptly serve.

For information about AtRandom.com Books and to sign up for our e-newsletters, visit www.atrandom.com.